Workers with Multiple Chemical Sensitivities

Mark R. Cullen, MD
Editor

Volume 2/Number 4 October–December 1987
HANLEY & BELFUS, INC.– Philadelphia

Publisher: HANLEY & BELFUS, INC.
210 South 13th Street
Philadelphia, PA 19107

OCCUPATIONAL MEDICINE: State of the Art Reviews is included in *Index Medicus*, *MEDLINE*, *Bio Sciences Information Service*, *Current Contents* and *ISI/BIOMED*.

OCCUPATIONAL MEDICINE: State of the Art Reviews   **(ISSN 0885-114X)**
October-December 1987   Volume 2—Number 4   **(ISBN 0932883-46-X)**

OCCUPATIONAL MEDICINE: State of the Art Reviews is published quarterly by Hanley & Belfus, Inc., 210 South 13th Street, Philadelphia, PA 19107. Second-class postage paid at Philadelphia, PA and at additional mailing offices.

POSTMASTER: Send address changes to OCCUPATIONAL MEDICINE: State of the Art Reviews, Hanley & Belfus, Inc., 210 South 13th Street, Philadelphia, PA 19107.

The 1988 subscription price is $64.00 per year U.S., $74.00 outside U.S. (add $24.00 for air mail). Single copies $29.00 U.S., $34.00 outside U.S. (add $6.00 for single copy air mail).

CONTENTS

IV. MANAGEMENT OF THE WORKER WITH MCS

PUBLISHED ISSUES

FUTURE ISSUES

Subscriptions and single issues available from the publisher—Hanley & Belfus, Inc., 210 South 13th Street, Philadelphia, PA 19107 (215) 546-7293.

CONTRIBUTORS

Carroll M. Brodsky, PhD, MD
Professor of Psychiatry, University of California, San Francisco, School of Medicine, San Francisco, California

Vera S. Byers, MD, PhD
Adjunct Associate Professor of Immunology in Dermatology, University of California, San Francisco, School of Medicine; Attending Physician, Moffett Hospital, San Francisco, California

James E. Cone, MD, PhD
Assistant Clinical Professor, University of California, San Francisco, School of Medicine; Chief, Occupational Health Clinic, San Francisco General Hospital, San Francisco, California

Mark R. Cullen, MD
Associate Professor of Medicine and Epidemiology, Yale University School of Medicine; Director, Yale-New Haven Occupational Medicine Program, New Haven, Connecticut

Leo Galland, MD
Private consulting practice, New York, New York

Robert Harrison, MD, MPH
Assistant Clinical Professor and Chief, Occupational and Environmental Medicine Clinic, University of California, San Francisco, School of Medicine, San Francisco, California

Stephen Michael Hessl, MD, MPH
Chairman, Division of Occupational Medicine, Cook County Hospital; Assistant Professor, Environmental and Occupational Health Sciences, University of Illinois School of Public Health, Chicago, Illinois

Alan Scott Levin, MD
Adjunct Associate Professor of Immunology in Dermatology, University of California, San Francisco, School of Medicine; Attending Physician, Moffett Hospital, Mt. Zion Hospital, and St. Mary's Hospital, San Francisco, California

Beth M. Lewis, MW, ACSW, CISW
Assistant Clinical Professor of Social Work in Medicine, Yale University School of Medicine; Social Worker, Yale-New Haven Hospital, New Haven, Connecticut

Robert Keene McLellan, MD, MPH
Assistant Clinical Professor of Medicine, Yale University School of Medicine, New Haven, Connecticut

Stephen B. Mooser, MPH
Program Administrator, Yale-New Haven Occupational Medicine Program, New Haven, Connecticut

Randy B. Reiter, PhD, MPH
Research Epidemiologist, University of California, San Francisco, School of Medicine; Occupational Health Clinic, San Francisco General Hospital, San Francisco, California

Richard S. Schottenfeld, MD
Assistant Professor of Psychiatry and Clinical Director, Substance Abuse Treatment Units, Yale University School of Medicine, New Haven, Connecticut

Judith Sparer, MSCE, CIH
Industrial Hygienist and Lecturer, Yale University Medical School, New Haven, Connecticut

Abba I. Terr, MD
Clinical Professor of Medicine, Stanford University Medical School; Consultant in Allergy, Letterman General Hospital, Courtesy Staff, St. Lukes Hospital, and Adjunct, Department of Medicine, Mt. Zion Hospital, San Francisco, California

PREFACE

"My dear friend," he would say, "I beg you: shall I be causing you much inconvenience if I ask you to take the handkerchief out of your jacket? You know how I can't bear any perfume. . . ."

And he gave three rings on the bell, out of habit, as if at his parents' house.

"Céleste, take the gentleman's handkerchief and put it in another room.—My dear friend, the last time you were so good as to come and see me—for nobody comes any more to see the wretched invalid that I am—I was obliged to take the chair you sat in and keep it out in the courtyard for three days: it was impregnated with the scent."

From *Marcel Proust: His Life and Work*,
by Léon Pierre-Quint, Peter Lang, 1925.

MARK R. CULLEN, MD

THE WORKER WITH MULTIPLE CHEMICAL SENSITIVITIES: AN OVERVIEW

The idea for this volume evolved from a stark and disconcerting clinical experience. Little more than a few months after the occupational medicine clinic began at Yale, in 1979, the staff was confronted with a problem none of us had ever seen before nor heard about. A middle-aged man was referred because of delayed recovery from an episode of pneumonia that had resulted from a chemical spill on the job. As his x-ray cleared, he had become not better, but worse. Particularly striking was the history that exposure to chemical odors would markedly exacerbate baseline dyspnea and chest pain. Upon return to work he "passed out" on several occasions after a whiff of fume. Disability leave, however, did not resolve the situation. Increasingly, even common household products and environmental contaminants induced debilitating respiratory and constitutional symptoms, reducing his formerly vigorous life to a pitiful existence at home. In response we exhaustively investigated his list of chemical precipitants in search for some way to tie these toxicologically with his prior pneumonia, but without success. Equally unrevealing were results of extensive clinical tests undertaken to define his "lesion" pathophysiologically. Therapeutically, it would be generous to say that we accomplished very little. There were other cases, too.

One day, a strident former machine operator came to the clinic wearing, much to everyone's amazement, a respirator. Suddenly, the image of the "gas mask" precipitated recognition of an identifiable clinical constellation, characterized by severe, recurrent and toxicologically inexplicable symptomatic reactions to quite low levels of common airborne substances. We discovered shortly that we were not alone. Many of our colleagues practicing occupational medicine around the country began reporting similar cases; they too were stymied by them. Thus we became aware of how widespread the problem is and how incredibly expensive the costs are for medical care and disability in each case.

Unfortunately, recognition of this "syndrome" did not lead readily to improved understanding nor to drastically enhanced therapeutic efficacy. To be sure, we were able in subsequent cases appropriately to abridge toxicologic investigation and to limit medical testing to areas where results were likely to have direct therapeutic benefit. In addition, we learned to avoid certain predictable pitfalls, such as extensive use of medications (which generally made patients worse) and projection of unrealistic expectations for rapid recovery after the almost invariably

From the Yale-New Haven Occupational Medicine Program, Department of Internal Medicine, Yale University School of Medicine, New Haven, Connecticut

Reprint requests to Mark R. Cullen, MD, Occupational Medicine Program, School of Medicine, 333 Cedar Street, New Haven, CT 06510

necessary step of removing the patient from his/her work environment. Furthermore, we began to recognize characteristic differences among patients, which
seemed to have some therapeutic value for certain groups, e.g., those meeting the
Diagnostic and Statistical Methods-III (DSM-III) standard psychiatric criteria for
post-traumatic stress disorder or variations thereof.[3,4] But on the whole, though
we were referred as many as one new patient monthly, neither our understanding
nor our approach substantially improved.

As we groped for some better conceptual framework, we became aware of the
considerable theoretical work in this area that had been generated by the movement
known as clinical ecology. Not only had some of our patients consulted these
specialists, but some clinical ecology precepts were gradually becoming incor-
porated into lay perceptions about chemicals and health; for example, not a few
of our clinic patients self-prescribed extensive dietary supplements of various kinds
for the treatment of every sort of occupational disease. The net effect was that we
were forced to confront these theories in practice, without proven alternative theories or treatments. Sadly, the existing literature on the subject was generally more
polemical than edifying.

It was to cope better with this situation that the staff of the Yale-New Haven
Occupational Medicine Program undertook the dialogue, both internally and with
investigators of varying perspectives throughout the country, that resulted ultimately in production of this volume. Like the proverbial blind men coming to know
the elephant, we began the process of sharing our perceptions, each with a particular slant or theory biased by experience.

Though we have not come a long way towards the goal of understanding the
problem, we felt that there might be some purpose at this time in summarizing
the current state of knowledge and opinion about these unfortunate and challenging
patients. We were well aware at the outset that the level of knowledge was slight,
the tenacity of opinions great and that those with differing views had long since
ceased serious dialogue or debate. It was our hope that by coalescing in a single
place existing thought we could hasten the only viable approach we know to such
a clinical problem—serious, open-minded scientific inquiry.

THE SYNDROME OF MULTIPLE
CHEMICAL SENSITIVITIES

Not least among the difficulties surrounding this subject, and certainly imped-
ing progress, is lack of uniform and appropriate nosology for atypical reactions to
chemicals. As discussed by several contributors to this volume, no fewer than a
dozen different names have been used by various clinicians and investigators,
each subtly or not so subtly implying a certain pathophysiologic basis or relationship
to other known disorders. Furthermore, as discussed briefly below, the diagnostic
"boundaries" that determine inclusion or exclusion from the various categories
differ widely, also reflecting very divergent views of the biology of the disorder(s).

In order to simplify, and hopefully clarify, matters, we chose to limit discussion as much as possible to a fairly narrow diagnostic grouping, which we have called multiple chemical sensitivities or MCS. While we felt this designation had inherent heuristic value, given current knowledge, we started this project with only a description of the disorder and some "exclusions"; we lacked a specific case definition. As the contributors responded, a pattern has emerged that can be roughly translated into a definition. We offer it here to clarify the focus of this volume and to spare the reader some of the confusion and difficulty with classification that has plagued the authors and editors (and the entire field):

Multiple chemical sensitivities (MCS) is an acquired disorder characterized by recurrent symptoms, referable to multiple organ systems, occurring in response to demonstrable exposure to many chemically unrelated compounds at doses far below those established in the general population to cause harmful effects. No single widely accepted test of physiologic function can be shown to correlate with symptoms.

Using this case definition, seven major diagnostic features can be distinguished:

1. *The disorder is acquired in relation to some documentable environmental exposure(s), insult(s) or illness(es).* This criterion restricts attention to patients who develop symptoms for the first time after some untoward encounter with their environment and specifically excludes patients with longstanding health problems who, later, may come to attribute certain symptoms to chemical exposure.

2. *Symptoms involve more than one organ system.* This limits attention to those patients with complex symptom patterns and eliminates, for example, patients with recurrent headaches or cough triggered by diverse stimuli.

3. *Symptoms recur and abate in response to predictable stimuli.* This excludes patients whose symptomatology is constant or has a pattern of variability largely unrelated to exposures.

4. *Symptoms are elicited by exposures to chemicals of diverse structural classes and toxicologic modes of action.* Individuals with classic allergic reactions to specific compounds and closely related substances, e.g., isocyanates or grains, are thus not included here.

5. *Symptoms are elicited by exposures that are demonstrable (albeit of low level).* By demonstrable we mean that people other than the patient should be aware of the chemical, e.g., smell it, even if not bothered by it. This criterion excludes frankly delusional patients and those who speculate (but cannot smell or otherwise define) that chemicals "must be present" whenever they feel poorly.

6. *Exposures that elicit symptoms must be very low, by which we mean many standard deviations below "average" exposures known to cause adverse human responses.* Since data on the range of "normal" responses are often unavailable, a rule of thumb would be that exposures are known to be generally lower than 1% of established threshold limit values (TLVs).

7. *No single widely available test of organ system function can explain symp-*

toms. This excludes, for example, individuals whose symptoms are attributable to bronchospasm, vasospasm, seizure disorder or any other reversible lesion that can be identified and specifically treated. Patients in whom symptoms alone can be provoked are not excluded, nor are those who may be shown to have an underlying biochemical or immunologic abnormality, unless associated *reversible* organ system function can also be shown.

THE RELATIONSHIP BETWEEN MCS AND OTHER "ENVIRONMENTAL" DISORDERS

Although the criteria listed should not be overly restrictive and describe a substantial patient population, there are obviously many patients meeting some but not all of them; several potentially relevant distinctions deserve mention.

First is the boundary between atypical variants of traditional "one-toxin" acute occupational diseases and MCS. For example, acute solvent intoxication certainly may occur in some individuals at exposure levels well below TLV's. As well, some cases of occupational asthma do not present to appropriate medical attention until bronchospasm has begun to occur in response to multiple, perhaps diverse, stimuli in addition to the initial offender. Yet however difficult the clinical problem of differentiation may be in a given case, there should be no logical overlap between these disorders and MCS. In MCS, every aspect of the relationship between the environment and symptoms has become generalized—multiple symptoms, multiple offending agents and ultra-low provoking doses. In traditional occupational diseases, the relationship between a non-trivial exposure to a single compound or chemical group and a unified complaint complex should be definable; any subsequent generalization must be physiologically explicable or attributed to a second process (e.g., a complication). Of course, it must be remembered that MCS itself may complicate some cases of "usual" occupational disease, so in that sense the categories may overlap. This relationship is depicted graphically in Figure 1.

The relationship between MCS and the class defined by clinical ecologists as "environmental illness" or "20th Century Disease" is more problematic. Probably ecologists would include every MCS patient in their somewhat larger category. On the other hand, we would exclude as MCS (by the definition above) patients with unclear or "masked" relationships between specific episodes of chemical exposures and subsequent symptoms. We have drawn this perhaps arbitrary distinction because without it the boundaries become far too ill-defined to allow intelligent discussion, let alone meaningful clinical studies. This is illustrated in Figure 2.

A third area in which distinction must be drawn is from the psychiatric perspective. Since by definition patients with MCS defy traditional diagnostic approaches and have recurring symptoms that are not readily explicable by available tests, most if not all will meet DSM-III criteria for some form of somatoform or psychosomatic illness. As we and others have demonstrated, some fulfill the

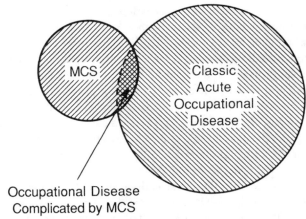

Figure 1.   Venn diagram of relationship between MCS and classic "one toxin" acute occupational diseases.

criteria for post-traumatic stress disorder or anxiety disorders.[1,3] Although these diagnoses may be technically correct, and indeed it may turn out (after careful clinical studies have been performed) that some or all MCS patients should be so classified, we would reserve for now these designations for those patients in whom the relationship between symptoms and environmental exposures is unclear, either

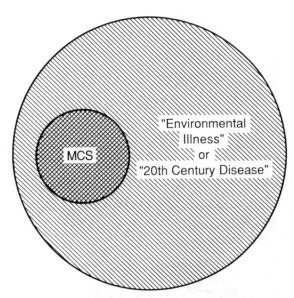

Figure 2.   Venn diagram depicting relationship between MCS and the designation "environmental illness" used by clinical ecologists. Inclusion in MCS requires a clear demonstration that symptoms are recurrent and predictably reproduced by actual environmental exposures.

because the symptoms long predate any awareness of environmental precipitants or because symptom variation is largely independent of objective environmental stimuli. Figure 3 depicts these relationships.

Two other important and recently recognized clinical syndromes in occupational medicine also deserve mention vis à vis MCS: tight building syndrome and mass psychogenic illness. In the tight building syndrome, now occurring in epidemic proportion in modern offices and other work places,[5] low levels of irritants combine with inadequate fresh-air intake and often low humidity to cause irritative symptoms often associated with CNS problems such as fatigue and poor concentration. Although all exposed workers may be affected, usually one or two are the most symptomatic, bringing the problem to light. For these "canaries," the differentiation from MCS maybe extremely difficult—in fact, these "index" cases may have or develop MCS in the course of discovery and resolution of the problem! The key to the distinction between tight building syndrome and MCS is in the epidemiology. In the former a clear pattern of dose-related symptoms will be elicited from the patient's co-workers. Furthermore, complaints are usually restricted to the single culpable environment at work and do not generalize as in MCS to other situations and substances.

Distinguishing MCS from the pattern of symptoms in workers suffering so-called mass psychogenic illness[2] may also be difficult, especially at first. In this disorder, symptoms of uncertain basis are believed to spread from an initially affected worker to others, leading to an outbreak; typical epidemiologic investigation fails to identify a pattern consistent with any toxic cause, so group psychological factors are invoked. As in the tight building syndrome, the index cases

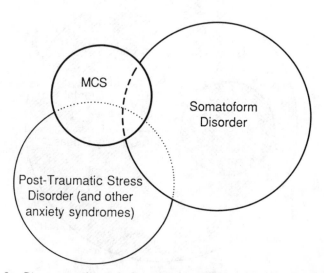

Figure 3. Diagramatic schema of relationship among MCS, somatoform illness and post-traumatic stress disorder (PTSD). The proportion of MCS patients who should correctly be classified as somatoform or PTSD remains a matter of speculation.

in such epidemics share features in common with MCS. The difference, once again, lies in the specific locale of complaints—the work environment—and the pattern of complaints in co-workers, however well toxicologically founded.

Having said all this, the reader should be reminded that the MCS designation with its above case definition is but one early attempt at a classification, chosen for its clinical usefulness given the current state of the art and for its potential usefulness in studies. Surely no strong inference can be made with present knowledge regarding a relationship or lack thereof between cases falling within this grouping and those sharing some, but not all, features. As noted above, even the biologic homogeneity and integrity of MCS itself is purely conjectural at present.

THE STRUCTURE OF THIS BOOK

In order to accomplish our purpose of bringing together in one place both a review of present data and a sampling of modern points of view, a dozen manuscripts were commissioned, about half from our own group, the remainder outside. The first paper, along with this introduction, addresses several issues germaine to the descriptive epidemiology of MCS and the syndromes with which it is most likely to be confused. As must already be evident from the classification difficulties, this area is sorely in need of more data.

The next three sections were designed to conform to a potential research agenda—pathophysiology, diagnosis and treatment, respectively. We realized quickly, however, that some present views are not organized easily along such conceptual lines; some chapters spilled a little. As clear reflections of the current level of discussion, there seemed little value in imposing our agenda on these exemplary contributions. Moreover, the considerable diversity of perspective becomes even more apparent when the relationships between scientific "theories" and clinical "facts" are explored. On the other hand, the book may be harder to use in some ways, since treatment for example, is discussed in more than double the three chapters Section IV might lead you to consult. Beware.

Finally, I want to personally thank everyone who participated in this effort, including those members of our faculty and staff who contributed to our thinking but not our writing. Special mention in this regard must be made of our colleague Dr. Laura Welch, now at George Washington, who never failed to challenge and improve our concepts about MCS during her years at Yale and thereafter.

REFERENCES

1. Brodsky CM: Allergic to everything: a medical subculture. Psychosomatics 24:731–42, 1983.
2. Colligan MJ, Pennebaker JW, Murphy LR (eds): Mass Psychogenic Illness. Hillsdale, NJ, Lawrence Erlbaum Assoc., Publ., 1982.
3. Schottenfeld RS, Cullen MR: Occupation-induced post traumatic stress disorders. Am J Psychiatry 142:198–202, 1985.
4. Spitzer RL (ed): Diagnostic and Statistical Manual of Mental Disorders, 3rd ed. Washington DC, Am Psychiatric Assoc., 1980.
5. Wadden RA, Scheff PA: Indoor Air Pollution. New York, John Wiley & Sons, 1983.

STEPHEN B. MOOSER, MPH

THE EPIDEMIOLOGY OF MULTIPLE CHEMICAL SENSITIVITIES (MCS)

> Much of our population is reacting adversely to the polluted air around us, the food we eat, the clothing we wear, the furniture we use, as well as to the medications we take. Our environment is rapidly becoming a threat to our physical, mental and emotional health. We are suffering from the "20th Century disease."[24]

> Many of the symptoms of 20th Century disease are characteristic of psychiatric disorders, but the patients resist psychiatric referral or treatment . . . Twentieth-century disease appears to be not a new illness but, rather, a fashionable name for a condition known to physicians for centuries.[17]

These statements mark the polarity of opinion and substantial debate over the existence and prevalence of environmental sensitivity.

In recent years, increasing attention has been directed toward the assessment of the impact of occupational and environmental exposures on human health. Amidst this process, a growing number of individuals and practitioners have raised concern about the possible adverse effects of many substances, even at low-level exposures.

This concern has generated increasing public involvement. For example, the Ministry of Health of the Province of Ontario, Canada commissioned a public policy study of environmental hypersensitivity which was completed in 1985. A year earlier, legislation to create an advisory committee on chemical hypersensitivity, which would have provided grants for research and education, passed both houses of the California legislature. The bill was vetoed, however, by Governor George Deukmejan.

The purpose of this chapter is to review available data regarding the epidemiology of "multiple chemical sensitivity" (MCS). This effort is confronted with a number of significant obstacles, not the least of which is the absence of a uniform definition of the condition itself.

Variously described as "environmentally-induced illness,"[1] "ecological illness,"[2] "food and chemical sensitivity,"[4] "chemical hypersensitivity syndrome,"[6] "Twentieth Century disease," or "total allergy syndrome,"[17] these designations allude to a group of individuals experiencing a constellation of symptoms perceived to be triggered by exposure(s) even to low levels of a variety of substances.

The search for a common definition, however, has been severely hampered

From the Occupational Medicine Program, Department of Internal Medicine, Yale University School of Medicine, New Haven, Connecticut

Reprint requests to Stephen B. Mooser, MPH, Occupational Medicine Program, Yale University School of Medicine, 333 Cedar Street, New Haven, CT 06510 by differences in terminology, the varied nature of the symptoms, the assessed degree of impairment, and controversy over diagnostic criteria. It is quite possible that among the patients described, there is not one single disorder but a number of different disorders with divergent underlying factors or combinations of factors (i.e., toxic exposures, auto-immunity, viral infection, fungal infection, endocrine dysfunction).

In its review of the definitions of this condition, the Committee on Environmental Hypersensitivity Disorders, commissioned by the Ontario (Canada) Ministry of Health, came to the following working definition:[13]

> Environmental hypersensitivity is a chronic (i.e., continuing for more than three months) multisystem disorder, usually involving symptoms of the central nervous system and at least one other system. Affected persons are frequently intolerant to some foods and they react adversely to some chemicals and to environmental agents, singly or in combination, at levels generally tolerated by the majority. Affected persons have varying degrees of morbidity, from mild discomfort to total disability. Upon physical examination, the patient is normally free from any abnormal objective findings.

PREVALENCE

As noted, the absence of common criteria and definitions makes quantification of individuals with multiple chemical sensitivities or any other related diagnostic group virtually impossible. The author could find no published estimates of prevalence among the general population. In conversations with some clinicians, estimates of those with substantive disruption of their lives due to MCS offered a range as high as 2 to 10% in the general population. The Ontario Canada Ministry of Health Report concluded:

> While we believe that there is evidence to support the view that a significant number of persons show symptoms of environmental hypersensitivity, we are unable to make any definitive statement about the prevalence of the disorder.[14]

MCS PATIENT PROFILE

Unfortunately, there also appears to be virtually no data published that characterizes the MCS population. Conversations with a number of clinicians do reveal, however, some common descriptions: a predominantly Caucasian female population in their 30s with an above average social-economic status (SES). Given the strong bias inherent with this condition to self-select treatment, coupled with the relatively high cost of treatment and its frequently disputed coverage by health insurance, few inferences can be drawn from the data that exists. Such data do tend to confirm informal observations and raise interesting questions worthy of further research.

The Committee on Environmental Hypersensitivity Disorders placed newspaper ads in 16 Ontario newspapers soliciting testimonials from individuals and organizations concerned about chemical sensitivity. Data were received from 130 individuals, representing 119 families, who characterized themselves as having MCS. Seventy-five percent of the respondents were female. The median number of years of symptomatology was eight. Primary systems reported as affected were the central nervous system (77%), respiratory system (45%) and gastrointestinal system (44%).[15]

The largest environmental control unit in the United States is located at Carleton Community Hospital in Carleton, Texas. The director of the program is William J. Rea, M.D. A review of 100 consecutive patients admitted to the environmental control unit in 1985 confirmed several of the informal observations mentioned earlier. The study population was 77% female, with a median age of 40. Race was not indicated. Of the group, 53.8% were highly educated, with 4 or more years of college. Most (56.3%) first experienced symptoms before they were 30 years of age.

When asked what they felt was the precipitating factor in the onset of their disease, 12% indicated occupational exposure to chemicals. Eleven percent specified a new environment (home, job, college). However, 58% were unable to identify a triggering set of circumstances. Less than half (42.9%) of those who reported exposure to chemicals on their job implicated such exposures as responsible for their illness.[19]

The most common finding in the limited available data is the predominance of females among MCS patients. While previous studies have established a higher level of reported symptomatology and physician utilization by female patients,[22] these findings do not adequately explain such a marked gender differential.

A number of studies have documented heightened drug allergies and food sensitivities among females, including such manifestations as eczema and hives.[5,7] Research has also indicated sex differences in enzyme and immune functions which may account for heightened allergic sensitivity.[9] Further study in this regard, as it applies to multiple chemical sensitivities, would be useful.

DIRECTIONS FOR THE FUTURE

Despite the virtual absence of epidemiological data, it has become increasingly evident to many occupational medicine clinicians around the country that there exists a not insignificant minority of patients with MCS. Whether this group is growing in number is not at all clear. It may be thought by some that this population is largely the creation of clinical ecologists, although this view does not seem to be confirmed by clinical histories. These histories often reveal extensive medical work-ups, frequently including psychiatric consultation, prior to evaluation by occupational medicine specialists or clinical ecologists.

While case reports cannot be considered reliable sources for confirmation of a diagnosis, they can provide useful direction in identifying areas worthy of research. The sheer volume and consistency of reports of individuals with chemical sensitivities is impressive and should be viewed as initial data in formulating research initiatives.

There are several factors that deserve further investigation and may provide insight into the prevalence of MCS. First, it is important to acknowledge the increased presence of a variety of chemical substances in our environment of which the acute and chronic effects have not fully been evaluated.

Recent evidence suggests a portion of the population is sensitive to quite low levels of environmental contaminants. In this regard, analysis of indoor air pollution, or tight-building syndrome, is instructive. This phenomenon has increased in the years following the institution of energy-saving measures, including "sealing" of buildings from natural ventilation. Through December 1985 the National Institute of Occupational Safety and Health (NIOSH) investigated 356 indoor air quality problems, primarily in government and private office buildings.

Inadequate ventilation was determined to be the primary cause of the problem in 50% of the investigations, while 30% were caused by either outside or inside contaminants.[23] While significant exposure levels were rarely found, complaints of eye irritation, dry throat, headache, fatigue, and sinus congestion occurred in a majority of the buildings investigated.

While some individuals have developed MCS following tight building syndromes, the overwhelming majority has not. The incidents are instructive, however, in that they provide evidence of the irritant effects of low-level exposures, as well as the variability of individual reactivity.

One of the common elements in case histories of individuals with MCS is adverse health effects from environmental exposure to perfume, fabric softener, cigarette smoke, etc. As indicated earlier, there are no estimates of the percentage of the population so affected. There is, however, evidence from a variety of arenas (i.e., increased incidents of indoor air pollution, legislative efforts to limit smoking in public and private facilities, the greater availability of unscented products) that such substances may be increasingly irritative to many in the general population.

Given well established principles of the variability of individual sensitivity to external stimuli, it is quite plausible that a subset of this group could exhibit reactions that go beyond irritation alone. Such reactions have not been reliably measured, although a recent study documented a decrement in pulmonary lung function among asthmatics when exposed to a variety of substances, including household cleaning agents, insecticides, perfume and cologne, and fresh paint smell.[16]

Research efforts are being focused on viral infections as a triggering factor in MCS. Adverse immunological impact from infection has been shown.[8,11] Until the recognition of acquired immune deficiency syndrome (AIDS), the potential for such immunological impact by a viral agent was not fully appreciated, nor were the reported symptoms of early AIDS victims uniformly considered to be physiological in nature. Recently, reports have indicated that the Epstein-Barr virus (EBV) can precipitate a persistent, chronic illness characterized by fever, fatigue, depression, paresthesia, mental confusion, psychoneuroses, headache, enlargement of liver or spleen, myalgia, and abdominal complaints.[21,10,12,18]

These research efforts are somewhat ancillary to what remains the primary controversy in the field: does MCS have a physiological basis(es) and, if it does, what triggers it. Clinical ecologists have developed several theories of hypersensitivity causation, i.e., total load, adaption, masking and bipolarity. (These theories are described in greater detail in the article by McLellan in this issue). Limited testing has been conducted to substantiate these theories. To date, experimental test support for these theories has been lacking, especially in the case of "masking" and "bipolarity." Clinical ecologists have come under fire for the dearth of reproducible, scientific research data substantiating immunologic impairment among MCS patients.[20]

In response to the development of the field of clinical ecology, a number of researchers have evaluated small subsets of affected individuals and concluded their symptomatology to be psychological in nature.[3,17,20] Principal criticisms of these studies, however, have included: (1) the difficulty of generalizing from small sample sizes; (2) the classification of individuals as exhibiting somatization disorder, which may reflect more on the problem than substantiate a diagnosis; and (3) the diagnosis of a psychological disorder that may be more the product of anxiety associated with chronic illness and the absence of diagnostic clarity than the causative disease factor.

Exploration of this phenomenon and the provision of high quality treatment for affected individuals are perhaps ill served by the focus and intensity of this debate. Indeed the complexity inherent in MCS may force us to question the usefulness of our reliance on the dominant paradigm of diagnosis, i.e., that causative factors are either physiological or psychological. It may also force us to humbly acknowledge the limits of our present knowledge of this field. The need for collaborative, multidisciplinary research to explore a host of possible causative factors is clear-cut. Such efforts may well lead to a more comprehensive understanding of MCS, one which may conclude that this condition is triggered by a combination of factors with no one factor uniquely significant in and of itself when examining the group as a whole.

In any event, it is incumbent to remember that after the debate about causative factors, there remains a population of infirm individuals who deserve our most competent and compassionate care.

CONCLUSION

Although the syndrome of multiple chemical sensitivities has received increasing attention in recent years, data concerning its prevalence among the general population is virtually non-existent. Lack of a common definition as well as the variability of symptoms and diagnostic criteria hamper this effort. Little data is available that characterizes the multiple chemical sensitive population, although incidence among females appears to be considerably higher. Further research is needed not only to better characterize the population but, more importantly, to evaluate potential triggering factors.

REFERENCES

1. American Academy of Environmental Medicine. Position Paper, 1984-85. Denver, Colorado, 1984.
2. Bell IR: Clinical Ecology: A New Medical Approach to Environmental Illness. Bolinas, California, Common Knowledge Press, 1982.
3. Brodsky CM: Allergic to everything: A medical subculture. Psychosomatics 24(8):731–742, 1983.
4. Crook WG: The coming revolution in medicine. J Tenn Med Assoc 76(3): 1983.
5. Eaton KK: The incidence of allergy—has it changed? Clin Allergy 12:107–110, 1982.
6. Environmental Health Association, Sacramento, California, 1985.
7. Eriksson NE, Formagen H, Svenonius E: Food hypersensitivity in patients with pollen allergy. 37:437–443, 1982.
8. Frik OL, et al: Development of allergy in children. I. Association with virus infections. J Allergy Clin Immunol 63:228–241, 1979.
9. Grossman CJ: Regulation of the immune system by sex steroids. Endocrine Rev 5:435–455, 1984.
10. Hamblin TJ, et al: Immunological reason for chronic ill health after infectious mononucleosis. Br Med J 287:85–88, 1983.
11. Joffe MI, et al: Lymphocyte subsets in measles. Depressed helper/inducer subpopulation reversed by *in vitro* treatment with levamisole and ascorbic acid. J Clinc Invest 72:971–980, 1983.
12. Jones JF, et al: Evidence of active Epstein-Barr virus infection in patients with persistent, unexplained illnesses: Elevated anti-early antigen antibodies. Ann Int Med 102:1–7, 1985.
13. Report of the Ad Hoc Committee on Environmental Hypersensitivity Disorders. Office of the Minister of Health, Toronto, Canada, 1985, pp 17–18.
14. Ibid, p 233.
15. Ibid, pp 121–142.
16. Shim C, Williams MH: Effect of odors in asthma. Am J Med 80:18–23, 1986.
17. Stewart D: Psychiatric assessment of patients with "20th Century Disease" ("total allergy syndrome"). Can Med Assoc J 133:1002–1006, 1985.
18. Straus SE, et al: Persisting illness and fatigue in adults with evidence of Epstein-Barr virus infection. Ann Int Med 102:7–16, 1985.
19. Study of 100 Consecutive Patients Admitted to the Environmental Control Unit at Northeast Community Hospital in Bedford, Texas. WJ Rea and Associates (unpublished).
20. Terr AI: Environmental illness: Review of 50 cases. J Allergy Clin Immunol 75:169, 1985.
21. Tobi M, et al: Prolonged atypical illness associated with serological evidence of persistent Epstein-Barr virus infection. Lancet I:61–64, 1982.
22. United States Department of Health and Human Services (PHS) No. 83–1572. Physician Visits: Volume and Interval Since Last Visit, June 1983; pp 16–17.
23. Wallingford K: NIOSH Industry Air Quality Investigations in Office Buildings. NIOSH, Cincinnati, Ohio, 1987.
24. Weiss L, Weiss M: How to Live with the New 20th Century Illness, 1983, p 1.

ALAN S. LEVIN, MD
VERA S. BYERS, PhD, MD

ENVIRONMENTAL ILLNESS: A DISORDER OF IMMUNE REGULATION

The massive increase in our environmental exposure to chemicals, both synthetic and natural, has altered our bodily makeup. It is now all but impossible to find an American that does not have a detectable level of synthetic chemicals like halogenated hydrocarbons in his or her body.[35] Environmental concentrations of natural chemicals such as ammonia and formaldehyde are many orders of magnitude higher than in the past. Humans have many biochemical scavenger systems that protect them from damage caused by chemically altered cells and proteins. However, since we are now exposed to much higher concentrations of natural chemicals, as well as massive amounts of synthetic chemicals to which our ancestors were never exposed, it is easy to see that, with regard to chemical exposures, our protective resources are taxed to a much greater extent than were theirs.

Intense exposure to high levels of toxic chemicals often causes cell death. The clinical symptomatology associated with this type of damage has long been recognized as the acute toxic effects of chemical exposure and has been well documented in the medical literature.[4,11,23,25,45,] Lately, physicians have become aware of the effects of chronic low-level exposure to toxic chemicals and their influence on the biologic regulatory mechanisms of the body. These factors serve as a foundation for the recognition of the disease called environmental illness.

In this chapter we would like to address the following issues:

1. What is the definition of environmental illness?
2. What is presently known about the pathophysiology of the illness?
3. How is the diagnosis made?
4. What are the etiological considerations in environmental illness?
5. How is environmental illness treated?
6. How can it be prevented?

DEFINITION

The term environmental illness is used to describe an acquired disease characterized by a series of symptoms caused and/or exacerbated by exposure to environmental agents. The triggering agents include industrial and domestic chemicals, cigarette smoke, diesel fumes, and alcoholic beverages. The symptoms

Reprint requests to Alan S. Levin, MD, 450 Sutter St., Suite #1138, San Francisco, CA 94108.

involve multiple organs in the neurologic, endocrine, genitourinary and immunologic systems. There is a large body of information documenting symptoms seen in individuals subjected to known acute or chronic exposure to given chemicals; the only truly novel aspect of environmental illness is the realization that similar symptom complexes frequently are seen in individuals without known "massive" exposure and the diagnosis can be make on the basis of these symptom complexes.

SIGNS, SYMPTOMS, AND LABORATORY FINDINGS

The more common symptoms are outlined as follows:

Neurologic: Patients report headaches, often migraine in nature.

Mental status changes mimicking a mild variant of Wernicke's encephalopathy are common. Patients describe a loss of short-term memory that is characterized by the need to carry paper for lists and notes, and inability to find their way to new destinations. They commonly describe going to a store and forgetting what they went to buy. They also describe dulling of cognition from smog and diesel fumes, such that they commonly miss familiar freeway exits while driving. People may also describe hearing their names called from a distant part of a quiet house when they are alone at home. Blood tests fail to show thiamine deficiency in these patients. Careful neuropsychological testing can identify various characteristics of this encephalopathy[7] that have previously been associated with exposure to certain chemicals.[15,58]

Visual anomalies mimicking migraine aura are common complaints. Patients see fleeting images in the periphery of the visual fields.

Peripheral neuropathies presenting as impairment or loss of peripheral sensation are often encountered. These can be documented on physical examination by loss of sharp/dull discrimination in the extremities and electromyographic (EMG) abnormalities. People whose jobs require fine motor control describe themselves as "clumsy." An increase in the number of falling accidents is seen in this population.[48] Acute loss of bowel or bladder control as a result of environmental exposure is another common complaint. Magnetic resonance imaging scans of the brain in such patients often show areas of increased signal intensity consistent with demyelination or microinfarcts.

Cardiac conduction system anomalies are commonly seen in this population. A 24-hour Holter monitoring reading demonstrates episodes of dysrhythmias when the patient is exposed to the triggering agent.[21,26,40,41,44,46]

Acquired alcohol intolerance is another common complaint. Patients who were previously able to tolerate alcoholic beverages commonly describe getting sick or drunk very quickly, often with a single mouthful of an alcoholic beverage.

Endocrine: Amenorrhea or dysmenorrhea is commonly found in females. Testing may demonstrate primary hypothalamic failure in these patients.

Fatigue and cold intolerance mimicking thyroiditis is another common complaint. Many such patients can be found to have anti-thyroid microsomal or thyroglobulin antibodies that often predate development of frank abnormalities in thyroid function tests. Occult thyroiditis is far more prevalent than previously thought.[14]

Fatigue, depression, and carbohydrate intolerance mimicking mild adrenal insufficiency is another common complaint. Cosyntropin stimulation tests not infrequently reveal minimal adrenal reserves in these patients.

Genitourinary: In addition to dysmenorrhea, there is a high incidence of miscarriages, congenital anomalies, and genitourinary tract disease requiring hysterectomy.[27] The incidence of cancer of the female reproductive tract is markedly increased in some populations.[27]

Immunologic: Chemically induced immune dysregulation is a recognized medical disorder.[23] A wide variety of symptoms referable to immune dysregulation can be seen in this population. Skin manifestations such as urticaria and induration are common. When exposure to toxic chemicals is through the GI tract, such as contaminated drinking water, perianal pruritis may be found.

Arthralgia with swelling but without morning stiffness is a common complaint. Rheumatoid factor is usually not detected on blood tests.

Chronic nausea with acquired food intolerance is a frequent complaint. This is a well recognized finding in chronic toxic chemical poisoning.[7,13] Food intolerance symptoms include all of the above mentioned nervous system symptoms, skin rashes, diarrhea, and bloating. Intradermal skin tests often confirm an immediate (IgE or IgG4) or a 24-hour delayed (IgG1 or 2) reaction to certain foods like milk, sugar, wheat, corn, and refined carbohydrates. Serial assessments of blood often show increased immune complexes associated with lowered complement components in response to ingestion of the suspect foods.[6,38]

Other symptoms referable to immune dysregulation include an increase in intensity of ordinary type 1 (IgE, IgG4-mediated) allergies and increasing sensitivity to body molds such as *Candida albicans* and Trichophyton. Mold allergy can manifest itself clinically as chronic dermatitis, gastroenteritis, and endogenous depression.[10,55]

Many patients respond inappropriately to viruses. This is manifested by the presence of the Epstein Barr early antigens (restricted and diffuse) long after the acute mononucleosis illness, presence of hepatitis B core antibody in the absence of hepatitis B surface antibody, indicating ongoing viral replication, and a protracted presence of IgM antibodies to the cytomegalovirus.[12,34] These patients have been classified by some physicians as suffering from a "chronic viral syndrome."[5,19,51] A large portion of this population can be found to have IgG subclass deficiencies.[36,51] Initial evidence of this state comes from the recognition that the adult patient with documented evidence of recurrent infections has a total IgG that is below the median for the expected range (1050 mg/dl). Subsequent measurement of IgG subclasses reveals a deficiency of one or more subclasses in a majority of these patients. Recent evidence suggests that some of this population suffers from infection with the Human B lymphocytotrophic virus (HBLV).[20,43,57]

Slight leukopenia is another common finding in these patients. Patients rarely have total white cell counts above 5500/cumm. Assessment of lymphocyte subpopulations often demonstrates low B cells and commonly shows low total T cells. Helper suppressor ratios are abnormal in a statistically significant number of these patients. These can be abnormally high or low, although the latter condition is more common. This is a reflection of an inordinately high number of suppressor cells rather than a diminution of helpers. This has led one investigator to postulate that these cells may be a population of natural killer cells that carry the CD 8 antigen (OKT 8, LEU 2) and are responding to a chemically transformed somatic cell.[9] Assessment of the data presented in a recent report appears to demonstrate these same findings, although the author concludes differently.[54]

A study of 78 females exposed to over 600 different chemicals in a computer manufacturing plant demonstrated substantial reduction of the helper/suppressor ratio as shown in Figure 1. When the exposed population was compared to the controls, the difference was statistically significant.[27] Notably, Hispanic female workers in this plant have a greatly increased incidence of cancer of the female reproductive tract when compared with age- and sex-matched controls.[27]

A representative group of individuals from a population exposed primarily to polychlorinated biphenols in their food chain and drinking water demonstrated similar abnormalities (Fig. 2). A statistically significant increase in the incidence

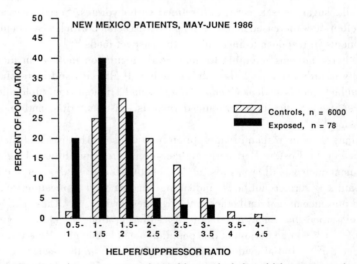

Figure 1. Helper/suppressor ratios obtained by standard clinical laboratory procedures on 78 injured workers from a computer chip manufacturing plant in Albuquerque, New Mexico compared with the standard laboratory control population of 6000 randomly selected asymptomatic people. The exposed population is statistically significantly different from the controls (chi-square = 39.34063; p = 2.62 × 10<−6>).[27]

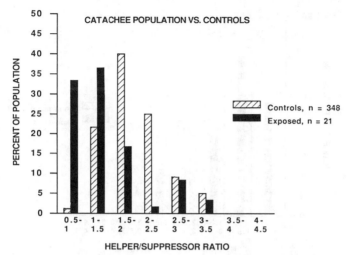

Figure 2. Helper/suppressor ratios obtained by standard clinical laboratory procedures on 21 environmentally ill patients who were domestically exposed to high levels of polychlorinated biphenols (PCBs) over a period of 5 to 10 years in Catachee, South Carolina, compared with the standard laboratory control population of 348 asymptomatic individuals. The exposed population is statistically significantly different from the controls (chi-square $= 63.48208$; $p = 1.37 \times 10 < -6 >$).[28]

of malignant melanoma and soft tissue sarcoma was demonstrated in this population.[29] A representative sample of a population of people exposed to trichloroethylkene and perchloroethylene in the city of Woburn, Massachusetts also demonstrated depression of helper/suppressor ratios (Fig. 3). A positive correlation between exposure to the contaminated water and leukemia was demonstrated in this population.[7]

A group of environmentally ill Wisconsin patients exposed to toxic chemicals in their drinking water also showed a depressed helper/suppressor ratio (Fig. 4).

Human population studies demonstrate an increased incidence lymphoreticular malignancy, soft tissue sarcoma, melanoma, and genitourinary tract cancer in individuals chronically exposed to similar chemicals.[18] Several recent population studies demonstrate immune aberrations associated with domestic exposure to toxic chemicals that are similar to those found as a result of industrial exposure.[16,39]

Reviewing the distribution of helper/suppressor ratios in exposed populations reveals a striking similarity in these parameters. This, along with the similarity in general medical symptomatology in these people, is evidence for a common pollutant as the cause of environmental illness.

HOW IS THE DIAGNOSIS MADE

Suspicion of environmental agents should be raised if a patient's symptoms have a strong neurologic component (encephalopathy and peripheral neuropathy),

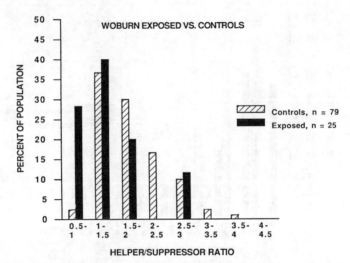

Figure 3. Helper/suppressor ratios obtained by standard clinical laboratory procedures on 25 environmentally ill patients from Woburn, Massachusetts who were domestically exposed to trichloroethylene (TCE) over a period of 5 to 10 years compared with age and sex matched asymptomatic controls.[7] The exposed population was statistically significantly different from the controls (chi-square = 42.18912; p = <1 × 10 <−8>). This control population is not significantly different from the standard laboratory controls used in the other studies.

evidence of immune system dysfunction (such as altered T- and B-cell functions and numbers), a history of recurrent infections (both bacterial and fungal), chronic skin rashes, arthritis or arthralgia, neoplasm (both benign and malignant), gastrointestinal symptomatology and/or cardiac dysrhythmias.

The diagnosis of environmental illness is made by history, physical examination, and laboratory testing. Patients may describe the abrupt onset of symptomatology associated with a specific insult. A typical comment of such an environmentally ill patient in this case is, "I have not been well since. . . ." The triggering event can be physical trauma such as an automobile accident, viral illness such as hepatitis or mononucleosis, or exposure to noxious chemicals. Patients may also describe a gradual onset of illness over a period of months or years. These patients commonly are found to have long-term low-dose exposures to toxins in the air or drinking water.

Individuals may respond differently to the same toxic substance. Therefore, a population of previously normal individuals that develops a panoply of multisystem complaints at the same time can be suspected of having environmental illness. Environmental assessment can often identify a causal factor.

When taking a history, care must be exercised to identify the circumstances of the patient's birth. Frequently individuals who experienced complicated pregnancies, such as maternal ingestion of prescription drugs (e.g., diethylstilbestrol

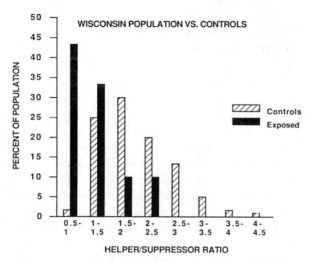

Figure 4. Helper/suppressor ratios obtained by standard clinical laboratory procedures on 10 environmentally ill patients from rural Wisconsin who were domestically exposed to a variety of industrial dyes, solvents, and pesticides over a 5 to 10 year period compared to the standard laboratory control of 6000 randomly selected asymptomatic people. The exposed are significantly different from the controls (chi-square = 73.58482; p = 4.77 × $10<-6>$).[30]

or recreational drugs and alcohol) are more susceptible to damage from environmental exposure to domestic and industrial chemicals. The patient's course during the common childhood viral illnesses of measles, mumps and chicken pox is an indicator of early immunologic problems. Measles or measles encephalopathy in childhood can be an indicator of diminished immune reserves in adulthood. Patients who have suffered more serious childhood viral illness such as polio and hepatitis are more susceptable to immune dysregulation as an adult. Some serious bacterial illnesses such as pertussis or pneumonias are associated with immune dysregulation in adult humans and animals.[24,47,56]

A patient's initial response to normal childhood vaccinations is important. Individuals who never developed an appropriate reaction to vaccinia ("smallpox take") may have longstanding T-cell defect. Individuals who developed severe arthus reactions to diphtheria-pertussis-tetanus vaccine may have longstanding immune dysregulation problem. A rather detailed chronologic history can uncover a history of multiple viral diseases, complications in a patient's childbearing history, physical traumas such as automobile accidents, and hospitalizations for other illnesses. A history of multiple surgeries requiring general anesthetics is important, since the patient's ability to tolerate such anesthetics is a clue to the presence or absence of environmental illness. Intraoperative anesthetic complications or serious difficulties recovering from the effects of the anesthetics are important historical considerations, since they indicate intolerance to synthetic chemicals.

ETIOLOGIC CONSIDERATIONS OF ENVIRONMENTAL ILLNESS

A causal agent in environmental illness is defined as a substantial contributing factor to the development of illness. If the patient were not exposed to this agent, he would not develop the disease at the same time and with the same intensity. To accurately identify a causal agent, one must first have objective evidence of the disease. This is obtained in routine fashion by history, physical examination, and laboratory testing. Often, laboratory testing of the entire exposed population shows a significant difference in the distribution of immune parameters when compared to controls. Therefore, testing simple immunologic parameters, such as B- and T-cell phenotypes with subset analysis, in the entire population can reduce the need to perform more elaborate testing in single individuals whose history and symptoms are consistent with a diagnosis but whose routine laboratory results are within the expected range.

The potential causal agent must be one that can realistically initiate an illness. If a patient whose history, physical findings, and laboratory results are consistent with a diagnosis of environmental illness described himself as completely well until he was exposed to the second-hand smoke of a single cigarette, another potential etiologic factor would be sought. If this patient described the onset of illness after a single exposure to an intensely toxic gas that is associated with severe acute symptoms, the toxic gas would be a candidate as the causal factor, since this is an etiologic agent that can reasonably cause disease.

WHAT IS KNOWN ABOUT THE PATHOPHYSIOLOGY OF THE ILLNESS

The symptoms of environmental illness are undoubtedly a result of numerous interactive biochemical phenomena. The biological regulatory systems—the interactive components of the neurologic, endocrine, and immunologic systems—are delicately balanced control mechanisms that involve the activity of many cells both to induce and to inhibit reactions. Like the servomechanisms in an autopilot, a series of counterforces maintains steady control. Health depends upon the appropriate balance of these forces. Agents that can alter this balance can cause diseases such as immune and endocrine dysregulation.

GROSS PATHOLOGY

Neurotoxic and irritant effects of chemicals produce direct pathological phenomena in target organs and may result in generalized immune and endocrine dysregulation. The medical literature is repleat with current references to the direct toxic effects of environmental agents on the neurologic and endocrine systems, as well as the more subtle secondary effects on target organs.[4,11,23,25,45] Since these subjects are so well covered in the existing medical literature, the gross pathological mechanisms of environmental illness will not be discussed here.

BASIC BIOCHEMICAL CONSIDERATIONS

The basic biochemical mechanisms by which toxic environmental agents cause damage can be divided into three major categories. These are quite similar to the effects of ionizing radiation:

Free Radical Generation and Alkylation. Toxic chemicals can cleave off electrons from proteins or cells, causing them to become highly reactive.[31,37] This causes the damaged moieties to become "glued" to other cells and proteins. As a result of this phenomenon, the function of the damaged protein or cell is altered. This can result in severe immunodeficiency.[8] In addition, these mechanisms trigger a series of immunologic phenomena.

Structural Alteration of Antigens. The alteration of tertiary structure in damaged cells and proteins causes them to become autoimmunogenic. This can result from the expression of previously hidden antigens (hidden epitopes). Such antigens are recognized by the natural immune mechanisms as senescent and attempts are made to remove them from the body.[22,32] Additionally, it has long been known that autoantibodies can be directed either to the primary or tertiary structure of antigens[3,52] and that the nature and severity of autoimmune disease is heavily influenced by these autoantibodies.[53]

Hapten/carrier Reactions. Environmental agents such as toxic chemicals can evoke immune reactivity by generating hapten/carrier reactions. Low-molecular-weight toxic chemicals, which alone are incapable of inducing an immune reaction, bind to larger molecules. This binding causes the small molecules to evoke an immune response. Subsequent exposure to the same or similar small molecule will cause a vigorous immune reaction.[1,2,17]

By these basic biochemical mechanisms, toxic environmental agents can both damage and tax the immune system at the same time. The damage can be both acute and cumulative. Since many toxic chemicals are lipophyllic and remain in the body for decades, their deleterious effects impact the health of an individual for long periods of time. It is easy to see why toxic chemicals can be more hazardous than ionizing radiation.

CLINICAL SYMPTOMATOLOGY AND IMMUNE COMPLEXES

As a clinician, one is struck with the similarity between the symptoms of environmental illness and acute infectious hepatitis patients. Fatigue, intolerance to alcohol and cigarette smoke, and multi-organ symptomatology are shared by those with environmental illness and hepatitis. Of importance is the fact that hepatitis does not become symptomatic until the patient has circulating immune complexes. Since immune dysregulation leads to immune complex disease, we investigated the possibility that an immune-complex-mediated, complement-consuming process could be partially responsible for the symptoms of environmental illness.[51] Upon evaluating a population of symptomatic patients, we discovered a significant number with elevated immune complexes (as measured by polyethylene glycol precipitation), depressed complement (as measured by C3) and elevated prostaglandin F2A, suggesting that part of their symptomatology was associated with an immune-complex-mediated inflammatory process.

HOW IS THE DISEASE TREATED?

The best treatment for environmental illness is avoiding the offensive agent. This can often be accomplished by simple environmental alterations, such as improving ventilation or wearing protective clothing and masks. Clinical improvement can often be accelerated by reducing the overall load on the immune system. This can be accomplished in most people with an allergy elimination diet. The diet is structured to remove the more common potential allergic offenders in an adult's diet. These include milk and milk products, cereal grains (wheat and corn), and refined carbohydrates (white sugar and white flour). A very common offender in individuals whose biological regulatory system has been damaged by environmental agents is the Candida albicans organism. This ubiquitous fungus is widely recognized as an allergen responsible for multi-organ symptomatology.[42] Oral administration of Nystatin (Nilstat) in large doses or careful administration of ketoconazole (Nizoral) can be very helpful. This treatment course has been described elsewhere.[10,55]

Specific antigen immunotherapy with ordinary allergy treatment for dust, grass pollens, molds, tree pollens, and weed pollens can be instituted to take the pressure off the damaged immune system. In refractory cases non-specific immunotherapy with transfer factor[29] and intravenous gammaglobulin has been found to be helpful. Transfer factor has been demonstrated to enhance both helper- and suppressor-cell activity,[29] while intravenous gammaglobulin provides the damaged immune system with idiotypic antibodies against various pathogens like virus, bacterium and fungus, as well as anti-idiotypic antibodies that reduce aberrant immune reactions.[49]

HOW CAN THE DISEASE BE PREVENTED?

Prevention is the most important and simplest aspect of this problem. First and foremost we must recognize the disease exists and that it is preventable. The simplistic explanation that it is conversion hysteria or malingering is untenable. Adequate ventilation of workplaces, utilization of appropriate protective clothing and respirators for workers, coupled with appropriate waste disposal techniques, will avoid contamination of workers and others with toxic chemicals and the spread of problems.

THE SOLUTION IS COMMON SENSE!

1. Try not to hurt anybody. Provide adequate ventilation, respirators, waste disposal, and medical screening to avoid toxic exposures.

2. If someone does get hurt, apologize by compensating him/her for their injury. Then alter the systems so that no one else gets hurt.

3. Recognize that people with environmental illness are genuinely made ill by noxious agents from the environment. It is unclear whether these people are just different in that they are more vulnerable or that they may be reacting in a more acute fashion to agents that also may, in the majority of the population, be responsible for otherwise unexplained chronic disease.

REFERENCES

1. Alkan SS, El-Khateeb M: Eur J Immunol 5:766–770, 1975 and Goodman JW, Fong S, Lewis GK, et al: Immunol Rev 39:36–59, 1978.
2. Alkan SS: Antigen recognition by T and B Cells: Studies with the azobenzene-arsonate-L-tyrosine system. *In* The Immune System, 2nd ed. (Basel Karger), 1981, pp 329–335.
3. Arana R, Seligmann M: Antibodies to native and denatured deoxyribonucleic acid in systemic lupus erythematosus. J Clin Invest 46:1867, 1967.
4. Asher IM (ed): Inadvertent Modification of the Immune Response: The Effects of Foods, Drugs, and Environmental Contaminants. Proceedings of The Fourth FDA Science Symposium, August 28–30, 1978. Superintendent of Documents, U.S. Government Printing Office, Washington, D.C. 20402.
5. Barnes DM: Mystery disease at Lake Tahoe challenges virologists and clinicians. Science 234:541–542, 1986.
6. Brostoff J: Immunoglobulin E receptors on inflammatory cells: the role of immunoglobulin E complexes in food allergy. Ann Inst Pasteur Immunol 137D:131–136, 1986.
7. Byers VS, Levin AS, Feldman R, et al: Clinical manifestations of a population with chronic domestic exposure to trichloroethylene (Ms. in preparation.)
8. Carson DA, Seto S, Wasson DB: Lymphocyte dysfunction after DNA damage by toxic oxygen species: A model of immunodeficiency. J Exp Med 163(3):146–151, 1986.
9. Colvin R: Personal communication, 1986.
10. Crook WG: The Yeast Connection, 3rd ed. New York, Random House Books, 1986.
11. Dean JH, Padarathsing M (eds): Biological Relevance of Immune Suppression As Induced by Genetic, Therapeutic and Environmental Factors. San Francisco, Van Nostrand Reinhold Co., 1981.
12. Dienstag JL, Wands JR, Koff RS: Acute hepatitis. *In* Petersdorf RG, et al (eds): Harrison's Principles of Internal Medicine, 10th ed. New York, McGraw-Hill Book Company, 1983, pp 1789–1797.
13. El Ghawabi SM, Mansoor MB, El Gamel MS, et al: Chronic trichloroethylene exposure. Egypt J Ind Med 715–724, 1984.
14. Ericsson U, Christensen SB, Thorell JI: A high prevalence of thyroglobulin autoantibodies in

adults with and without thyroid disease as measured with a sensitive solid-phase immunosorbent radioassay. Clin Immunol and Immunopath 37:154–162, 1985.

15. Feldman RG, White RF, Travers PH: Adverse health effects of pollutant exposure: Neurobehavioral disorders. Tarcher OR (ed): Principals and Practice of Environmental Medicine. New York, Plenum Press. In press, 1986.

16. Fiore MC, Anderson HA, Hong RA, et al: Chronic exposure to aldicarb-contaminated groundwater and human immune function. Environ Res 41:633–645, 1986.

17. Goodman JW, Fong S, Lewis GK, et al: Immunol Rev 39:35–59, 1978.

18. Hoar SK, Blair A, Holmes FF, et al: Agricultural herbicide use and risk of lymphoma and soft-tissue sarcoma. JAMA 256(9):1141–1147, 1986.

19. Jones JF, et al: Evidence for active Epstein-Barr virus infection in patients with persistent unexplained illnesses: elevated anti-early antigen antibodies. Ann Intern Med 102:1, 1985.

20. Josephs SF, Salahuddin SZ, Ablashi DV, et al: Genomic analysis of the human B-lymphotropic virus (HBLV): Science 234:601–603, 1986.

21. Kalsner S, Richards R: Coronary arteries of cardiac patients are hyperreactive and contain stores of amines: A mechanism for coronary spasm. Science, March 30, 1984, pp 1435–1437.

22. Kay MMB: Aging of cell membrane molecules leads to appearance of an aging antigen and removal of senescent cells. Gerontology 31(4):215–235, 1985.

23. Koller LD: Effect of chemical sensitivity on the immune system. Immunology and Allergy Practice 7(10):405–417, 1985.

24. Kong AS, Morse SI: The Effect of bordetella-pertussis on the antibody response in mice to type III pneumococcal polysaccharide. J Immunol 116(4):989–993, 1976.

25. LaDou J (ed): Occupational Medicine: State of the Art Reviews. The Microelectronics Industry. Philadelphia, Hanley & Belfus, Inc., January, 1985.

26. Levi R: Sudden death—an allergic reaction? Presented at 56th Scientific Sessions of the American Heart Association, 1983.

27. Levin AS: Presented in Romero AC, et al vs. GTE, Second Judicial District Court, New Mexico, CV-84-06943, 1984.

28. Levin AS: Presented in Whitfield C vs. Sangamo, Federal Court, Catachee, So. Carolina 8:84–3184–3, 1984.

29. Levin AS: Transfer factor therapy in food allergies. Brostoff J, Challacombe L (eds): Food Allergies. London, Tindall-Saunders Books, 1987, pp 995–1004.

30. Levin AS: Presented in Shiesel, et al and Hagen ON vs. Uniroyal, Inc., Circuit Court, Dane County, Wisconsin 83-CV-1116, 1983.

31. Levine SA, Kidd PM: Antioxidant Adaptation. Biocurrents Division, Allergy Research Group, San Leandro, CA, 1985, pp 236–245.

32. Lutz HU, Flepp R, Strigaro-Wipf G: Naturally occurring autoantibodies to exoplasmic and cryptic regions of band 3 protein, the major integral membrane protein of human red blood cells. J Immunol 133(5):2610–2618, 1984.

33. McGovern JJ, Jr, Lazaroni JL, Saifer, et al: Clinical evaluation of the major plasma and cellular measures of immunity. Journal of Orthomolecular Psychiatry 12:1–8, 1983.

34. Meyers JD: Cytomegaloviral infections. In Petersdorf RG, et al (eds): Harrison's Principles of Internal Medicine, 10th ed. New York, McGraw-Hill Book Company, 1983, pp 1167–1170.

35. Nader R, Brownstein R, Richard J: Who's Poisoning America. San Francisco, Sierra Book Clubs, 1981.

36. Oxelius V-A, Linden V, Christensen KK, Christensen P: Deficiency of immunoglobulin G subclasses in mothers of infants with group B streptococcal septicemia. Allergy Appl Immunol 72(3):249–252, 1983.

37. Padarathingh ML, Dean JH, Keys L: Effects of alkylating agents on the immune response. In Biological Relevance of Immune Suppression as Induced by Genetic, Therapeutic and Environmental Factors. San Francisco, Van Nostrand Reinhold Co., 1981, pp 176–189.

38. Pagnelli R, Levinsky RJ, Brostoff J, Wraith DG: Immune complexes containing food proteins in normal and atopic subjects after oral challenge and effect of sodium cromoglycate on antigen absorbtion. Lancet 1(8129):1270–1272, 1979.

39. Pross HF, Day JH, Clark RH, Lees REM: Immunologic studies of subjects with asthma exposed to formaldehyde and urea-formaldehyde foam insulation (UFFI). J Allergy Clin Immunol 79:797–810, 1987.

40. Rea WJ: Environmentally triggered cardiac disease. Ann Allergy 40:243–251, 1978.

41. Rea WJ: Review of cardiovascular disease. In Frazier CA: Bi-Annual Review of Allergy, 1979–1980, pp 282–347.

42. Rippon JW: Medical Mycology, 2nd ed. Philadelphia, W. B. Saunders, 1982, pp 507–508.
43. Salahuddin SZ, Ablashi DV, Markham FD, et al: Isolation of a new virus, HBLV, in patients with lymphoproliferative disorders. Science 234:596–600, 1986.
44. Seyal AR: Polyester PVCs. Indian Heart J 36:1, 1984.
45. Sharma RP: Immunologic Considerations in Toxicology, I & II. Boca Raton, FL, CRC Press, 1986.
46. Shimokawa H, Tomoike H, Nabeyama S, et al: Coronary artery spasm induced in atherosclerotic miniature swine. Science 221:560–561, 1983.
47. Schwab JH: Suppression of the immune response by microorganisms. Bacteriol Rev 39(2):121–143, 1975.
48. Small BM: Environmental Health Factors in Falling Accidents. Research undertaken under DSS Contract #05SX 3115-2-3205 for the Medical Engineering Section, Division of Electrical Engineering, National Research Council of Canada, Ottawa, Ontario Canada K1A OR6.
49. Stampf JL, Castignoli N, Epstein WL, Byers VS: Transfer of tolerance to mice by IgG from humans desensitized to poison oak. Ms. submitted, 1987.
50. Stanley PJ, Corbo G, Cole PJ: Serum immunoglobulin G subclasses in chronic and recurrent respiratory infections. Clin Exp Immunol 58(3):703–708, 1984.
51. Straus SE, et al: Persisting illness and fatigue in adults with evidence of Epstein-Barr virus infection. Clin Exp Immunol 58:7, 1984.
52. Tan EM, Schur PH, Carr RI, Kunkel HG: Deoxyribonucleic acid (DNA) and antibodies to DNA in the serum of patients with systemic lupus erythematosus. J Clin Invest 45:1732, 1966.
53. Tan EM, Rothfield NF: Systemic lupus erythematosus. *In* Sampter M (ed): Immunological Diseases. Boston, Little, Brown, 1978, pp 1038–1060.
54. Terr AI: Environmental illness, A review of 50 Cases. Arch Intern Med 146:145–149, 1985.
55. Trowbridge JP, Walker M. The Yeast Syndrome. New York, Bantam Books, 1986.
56. Vogel FR, Klein TW, Stewart WE II, et al: Immune suppression and induction of gamma interferon by pertussis toxin. Infect Immun 49(1):90–97, 1985.
57. Weiss R, Mulder C: A new human herpesvirus. Nature 323:762, 1986.
58. White RF: The role of neurologic testing in the evaluation of toxic CNS disorders. Seminars in Occupational Medicine 1:191–196, 1986.

ABBA I. TERR, MD

"MULTIPLE CHEMICAL SENSITIVITIES:" IMMUNOLOGIC CRITIQUE OF CLINICAL ECOLOGY THEORIES AND PRACTICE

The theories and practice of clinical ecology are having an increasing impact on occupational medicine. Claims of occupational disease diagnosed as "environmentally induced illness" or "chemical hypersensitivity syndrome" emanating from a small group of physicians identifying themselves as clinical ecologists are a source of confusion and concern not only to physicians and other health professionals, but to all those concerned with the health and safety of workers. Clinical ecology has recently been the subject of a position statement by the American Academy of Allergy and Immunology[2] and of a scientific investigation by the California Medical Association.[4]

This article is a critical review of clinical ecology as seen by an immunologist. Relevant articles from the clinical ecology literature dealing with its history, theory, and practice will be reviewed as they relate to immunology.

HISTORY OF THE CLINICAL ECOLOGY MOVEMENT

Clinical ecology is an alternative form of medicine practiced by several hundred physicians in North America and Great Britain. Its influence in medical practice of other countries is probably minimal. The movement evolved from clinical allergy, although its practitioners today are drawn from those who previously practiced in a variety of medical, surgical, pediatric, and psychiatric specialties. Clinical ecology is not taught in any American medical school, but its methods and theories may be learned from postgraduate courses and apprenticeships.

The origins of clinical ecology appeared in the 1930s and 1940s when Rowe, Randolph, and Rinkel expanded the concept of food allergy to include a causative role for it in chronic diseases of unknown etiology, such as rheumatoid arthritis, ulcerative colitis, and migraine. They also proposed food allergy as a cause of common nonspecific symptoms such as headache, muscle and joint aching, fatigue, depression, irritability, hyperactivity, and functional gastrointestinal disorders.[27-29] In 1954 Speer introduced the term "allergic tension-fatigue syndrome" to denote the belief that allergy to foods and inhalants caused behavioral and cognitive symptoms in patients without atopic manifestation.[31]

From Division of Immunology, Stanford University Medical School, Stanford, California

Reprint requests to Abba I. Terr, MD, Division of Immunology, Stanford University Medical School, Stanford, CA 94305

In the early 1950's Randolph introduced the idea that synthetic chemicals in the environment were similarly responsible for a wide variety of symptoms and that a pathological process in such patients was initiated by an environmental chemical exposure.[17,18] This idea led to a proposed new disease and the subject of this volume: multiple chemical sensitivities.

Clinical ecologists today continue to emphasize the importance that they attribute to foods and chemicals in causing symptoms, but in recent years they have added endogenous hormones and the ubiquitous yeast, *Candida albicans*,[7] to the list of items responsible for this disease.

ENVIRONMENTAL ILLNESS

"Environmentally included illness" or "chemical hypersensitivity syndrome" are the names most frequently used to designate the disease diagnosed and treated by clinical ecologists. A variety of other names have been applied to this illness (see Table 1). Environmental illness will be the term used in this review. There is no concise definition of environmental illness in the clinical ecology literature. A committee of the Ontario Ministry of Health after interviewing clinical ecologists and their patients established their own definition:

> Environmental hypersensitivity is a chronic (i.e., continuing for more than three months) multisystem disorder, usually involving symptoms of the central nervous system. Affected persons are frequently intolerant to some foods and they react adversely to some chemicals and to environmental agents, singly or in combination, at levels generally tolerated by the majority. Affected persons have varying degrees of morbidity, from mild discomfort to total disability. Upon physical examination, the patient is normally free from any abnormal, objective findings. Although abnormalities of complement and lymphocytes have been reported, no single laboratory test, including serum IgE, is consistently altered. Improvement is associated with avoidance of suspected agents and symptoms recur with reexposure.[5]

This statement does not define a disease. It merely restates the wide-ranging subjective complaints that clinical ecologists and their patients believe are caused by foods and environmental chemicals.

TABLE 1.   Environmental Illness: Synonyms

Environmentally-induced illness
Chemical hypersensitivity syndrome
Complex allergy
Cerebral allergy
Chemically-induced immune dysregulation
Twentieth century disease
Total allergy syndrome
Ecologic illness
Allergic toxemia
Environmental hypersensitivity disorder

Dickey defines ecologic illness as "an adverse reaction to environmental insult or excitant in air, water, food, drugs, or our habitat—domiciliary, occupational, or avocational."[9] This statement fails to identify the clinical manifestations of the disease, although it does emphasize the unlimited sources and nature of the presumed environmental causes.

A study undertaken specifically to define and characterize the clinical history, physical findings and laboratory abnormalities in patients with a diagnosis of environmental illness showed that—even in retrospect—the illness defies definition.[32] The most common complaints—fatigue, headache, nausea, malaise, pain, mucosal irritation, disorientation, and dizziness—are nonspecific and do not suggest organ system dysfunction. The absence of objectively verified abnormalities detected by physical examination, specific organ functioning, or laboratory testing means that the illness is subjective only. To date no gross or microscopic evidence of inflammation or other pathology for this disease can be found in the clinical ecology literature.

DIAGNOSIS OF ENVIRONMENTAL ILLNESS

Clinical ecology diagnosis is based on history, elimination diets, and several varieties of provocation testing. Particular emphasis is placed on the history and results of provocation tests, but little if any attention is paid to physical findings. Certain immunological tests on blood samples are used by some clinical ecologists in diagnosis.

The history taken by clinical ecologists stresses the patient's assessment of environment in the production of symptoms. An extensive questionnaire is usually used as an adjunct to the clinical ecologist's history. The questionnaire typically emphasizes details of the patient's diet and exposure to airborne substances at home and at work. Patients are encouraged to recall what was eaten, touched, or smelled prior to each exacerbation of symptoms. A unique feature of clinical ecology history is the lack of specificity of symptoms, i.e, any subjective complaint can be included in arriving at the diagnosis, even if these complaints are more likely caused by a non-environmental illness.[32] Some patients carrying the diagnosis of environmental illness are asymptomatic.

Objective physical findings play little if any role in diagnosis. In fact clinical ecology textbooks make no mention of physical examination in diagnosis.[3,9] The disease process is perceived as polysymptomatic with little if any objective loss of bodily functions or anatomic abnormality.

Major emphasis is placed on provocation testing for diagnosis. Three testing methods are generally used: intradermal provocation-neutralization, sublingual provocation-neutralization, and the use of airborne exposures to chemical fumes in special environmental control facilities. In each case a positive test result is indicated by the appearance of subjective symptoms. Occasionally physical findings or laboratory tests are reported as part of the challenge procedure.

Intradermal provocation-neutralization is performed by injecting intradermally different volumes (usually 0.01 or 0.05 ml.) of varying dilutions of test substances. The test substances most commonly include aqueous extracts of foods, food additives, inhalant allergens, "chemicals" (e.g., formaldehyde, phenol, ethanol, glycerine), "hormones" (e.g., progesterone, estrogen), histamine, tobacco, newsprint, saline, and water. Tests are performed one at a time. The patient records all symptoms and sensations during the ten-minute period following injection. The appearance of *any*, symptom constitutes a positive test, i.e., a state of hypersensitivity to the test substance. If there are no symptoms, progressively higher doses are administered until there is a positive response. Next, a lower dose is given, and if no symptoms are elicited during the ten-minute test period, this dose is designated as a "neutralizing dose." Self-administered injections at the neutralizing dose are then used by the patient as a form of therapy to "neutralize" symptoms. Symptoms that qualify as a basis for a positive test during provocation-neutralization need not be the same ones as those elicited by the history.

The sublingual provocation-neutralization procedure is identical except that the test dose is delivered by sublingual drop. The same test substances, timing, and symptom-reporting methods are used. There are reports of positive reactions to extremely minute quantities of foods or chemicals by this method. For example, in one reported case[26] the patient responded to one drop of kerosene diluted in saline by a factor of 5^{15} and to 0.4% phenol diluted 10.[15]

Several "environmental control units" for diagnostic testing are in operation in the United States. One such unit has been described as free of fumes and particles through the use of special construction materials, heating, lighting, and air filtration. No plastic furnishings or synthetic fabrics are permitted in the unit, since it is used to test patients believed to be exquisitely sensitive to ultra-low levels of environmental chemicals. The patient is exposed in special rooms to the fumes of such items as natural gas flame, cigarette smoke, perfume, Pine-Sol, ethanol, synthetic clothes, and carpets.[24] As in provocation-neutralization testing any symptom constitutes a positive response. No standards have been established for the concentration of material used for testing or for the duration of exposure.

Elimination diets and oral food challenges are also used by clinical ecologists for diagnosing sensitivity to foods. In some cases elimination of "highly allergenic foods" for a period of several days—usually one week—is followed by daily single-food challenges to elicit symptoms. Some practitioners have the patient fast for up to five days prior to challenge. Foods purchase in "organic" food stores are preferred for testing, since they are believed to be free of pesticide residues and additives. As in chemical testing, the appearance of subjective symptoms is the criterion for diagnosing sensitivity to foods. Some patients are said to be sensitive to tap water or spring water, presumably from naturally occurring or deliberately added chemicals.

Clinical ecologists will occasionally monitor blood pressure, nasal congestion, pulmonary function, handwriting, drawing ability, and psychological responses as part of the provocation test. Electrocardiogram[25] and electroencephalogram[6] changes have been reported. Practitioners who use intradermal provocation testing will sometimes, but not routinely, include an increase in size of the skin wheal at the test injection site as evidence of sensitivity. Changes in immunological tests will be discussed below.

TREATMENT OF ENVIRONMENTAL ILLNESS

Clinical ecology treatment utilizes three modalities: avoidance of environmental chemicals, elimination diets, and symptom neutralization. Drugs are generally avoided, since they are classed as synthetic chemicals and therefore disease-producing, although some clinical ecologists recommend the use of vitamin and mineral supplements.

Avoidance is the linchpin of therapy. Specific recommendations vary according to the enthusiasm of the individual practitioner and patient. The aim appears to be the achievement of a natural environment through elimination of "toxic" and synthetic chemicals. Substances to be avoided usually include perfumes, cosmetics, deodorants, synthetic clothing, soft plastics, carpets, and solvents. Specific chemicals most often mentioned as harmful and therefore to be avoided are formaldehyde, ethanol, phenol, and "petrochemicals" in general. The actual procedure for carrying out the recommended avoidance of environmental chemicals depends upon the patient's financial resources and perception of the illness. Some simply eliminate scented products, whereas others resort to extensive reconstruction of the home or a move to a less inhabited area such as a mountain community or seashore. In many cases the illness generates a claim of work disability.[32] Groups of patients have banded together into communities or trailer parks. Certain homes have been designated as "safe houses."

Lack of symptomatic improvement from these environmental avoidance measures—or the return of symptoms after temporary relief—are taken as a sign that additional eliminations are necessary. Clinical ecologists believe that some of their patients become ill from exposure to ordinary ambient levels of airborne chemicals unmeasurable by any existing method, and they have proposed that such persons could serve as a biological monitor for detection of exceedingly low levels of environmental chemicals.[24] The elimination diet is an essential component of the overall avoidance program. The list of specific foods to be eliminated is based on the patient's history and results of provocation-neutralization testing. In many cases the number of symptom-provoking foods is so great that complete elimination is incompatible with proper nutrition, so a "rotary diversified diet" is prescribed, whereby each food in the diet is eaten at intervals of four or five days.[28] Chemical food additives are avoided completely by shopping in health food stores. Some practitioners feel that tap water is unhealthy and they recommend bottled spring water.

In addition to avoidance of chemicals and foods, most patients are prescribed neutralization therapy, whereby subcutaneous and/or sublingual (occasionally intracutaneous) administration of "antigens" is used to treat or prevent symptoms. "Antigens" consist of extracts of foods, chemicals, hormones, atopic allergens, and even autocoids such as histamine, heparin, and serotonin. Subcutaneous injections or sublingual drops are self-administered on a regular daily schedule when symptoms appear, or they are used prior to anticipated exposure. Selection of substances for neutralization are likewise based on history and provocation testing. Symptom relief is expected to occur immediately.

IMMUNOLOGIC THEORIES IN CLINICAL ECOLOGY

The clinical ecology literature provides several theories to explain environmental illness. Immunologic mechanisms are prominent in these theoretical formulations.

Randolph's proposal that symptoms of intolerance to certain chemicals are caused by a failure in adaptation of the body to an unnatural (i.e., artificially synthesized) chemical is an extension of Selye's General Adaptation Syndrome. [19,30] Selye viewed the endocrine organs, especially the pituitary-adrenal axis, as a alarm system reacting to external stimuli. Continued stimulation was thought to lead to a phase of adaptation followed by a phase of exhaustion and thereby to the production of disease. [30]

Clinical ecologists regard disease as synomous with symptoms. Rea suggested that the mechanism for exhaustion or failure of internal homeostasis may be an immunologic one, in which environmental chemicals function as haptens, thereby inducing IgG antibodies. [26] The formation of circulating immune complexes in turn would activate complement to generate mediators of inflammation. He suggested as an alternative mechanism that these same chemicals might induce autoantibodies to blood vessel antigens causing vasculitis in some patients. [23] It was further postulated that individual susceptibility to disease was caused by a defect in certain enzyme systems, linked in some way to inappropriate function of the immune system.

Rea[25] and other clinical ecologists believe that environmental chemicals disturb the normal process of immune regulation, thereby causing either IgE-mediated release of mast cell mediators or IgG-mediated complement activation and immune complex formation. The environmental chemical therefore is an immunotoxin rather than an immunogen, according to this theory.

McGovern, et al. have extended this idea further by stating that it is "commonly understood that the T suppressor cell is more sensitive to damage from chemicals and other agents that are T helper cells."[16] Patients with environmental illness should therefore have a higher than normal ratio of T helper cells to T suppressor cells. According to this theory, the abnormally high ratio would stimulate an enhanced B cell activity leading to excessive antibody production and a hypersensitive state.

A somewhat different approach is taken by Levine, et al. who speculate that environmental illness is a manifestation of inflammatory mediators released from lipid peroxidation of cell membranes, initiated not by an immune reaction but rather by a toxic effect of free radicals generated by environmental chemicals, drug metabolites, and certain foods. [13] In this theory individual susceptibility results from a deficiency of normal antioxidants. The effects of free radical oxidation are said to include immunosuppression, autoimmunity, diminished resistance to infection, and "chemical allergy."

All of these various immunologic theories embrace a concept of "total body load" in which the immune system is likened to a barrel able to hold only a limited quantity of antigen from foods, from synthetic chemical additives in food and water, and from air pollutants. Symptoms result when antigen overexposure causes the barrel to overflow. This might occur from either a single massive overexposure or through chronic daily contact with ordinary concentrations of chemicals and/or foods. Physiologically the "barrel" is a metaphor for the macrophage, which presumably spills immune complexes into the circulation when overloaded with environmental antigens.[26]

IMMUNOLOGIC FINDINGS IN ENVIRONMENTAL ILLNESS

Data from the clinical ecology literature supporting an immunopathogenesis for environmental illness are limited to several articles comparing the patient's circulating immunoglobulin levels, complement components and blood lymphocyte counts to normal laboratory reference ranges. Rea states that serum concentrations of immunoglobulins are normal, C3 moderately reduced, and C4 elevated in this disease, but no data are presented.[23] In ten patients with "environmentally-induced thrombophlebitis," C4 is reported to be elevated in all, IgE "normal to low", and IgG and C3 usually normal.[22] In 12 patients with environmental sensitivity IgG was low in several, CH100 low in nine, C3 low in nine, and C4 high in five.[26] Selected patients from that report were described as having changes in circulating levels of T cell counts, IgG, eosinophil counts, and total complement with either challenge or avoidance, but the reproducibility of these changes with rechallenge was not established. There were no controls using similar challenges in unaffected subjects. Rea discussed 12 patients with environmentally-caused cardiac disease who had normal immunoglobulins, but total hemolytic complement and C3 were decreased and C4 increased in several of the patients.[25] Immunologic data from a 124 patients with "food allergy and phenol intolerance" showed some abnormal values, but these were not analyzed statistically.[16] Some abnormalities were exactly opposite those previously reported—for example, elevated total complement and reduced C4. The effect of oral challenge with foods or inhalation challenge with chemicals in selected patients produced a variety of changes in serum immunoglobulins, lymphocyte counts, complement components, and inflammatory mediators but only in some of the cases.[15] Many of the "changes" were within normal limits, and there were no consistent trends within the entire test group. In the three reports of immunologic changes induced by food or chemical challenge, two employed no controls,[16,26] and in the third study the control values, said to be "essentially normal," were not given.[15] Reproducibility of results was not established in any of these studies.

DISCUSSION

Critical analysis of the claim that environmental illness is an immunologic disorder requires an examination of (1) the clinical features, (2) pathology, (3) theories of immunopathogenesis, (4) laboratory evidence of immunopathology, (5) diagnostic testing methodology, and (6) the course of the disease including response to clinical ecology treatment.

CLINICAL MANIFESTATIONS OF ENVIRONMENTAL ILLNESS

The disease is presented as one with multiple symptoms and no consistent physical findings. Early reports by clinical ecologists indicate that they were attempting to identify a physical—i.e., environmental—cause for the multisystem complaints of patients with psychosomatic illness.[21] Subsequently patients with organ-specific symptoms, such as those involving cardiovascular,[23,25] behavioral,[12,18] gastrointestinal, and genitourinary complaints[8] have been included in the environmental disease picture. Even some patients with no symptoms whatsoever have been diagnosed as having environmental illness.[32] Clinical ecologists emphasize the often bizarre, variable, and wide-ranging complaints of their patients,[3] and they include other recognized diseases such as asthma, migraine, bronchitis, and various forms of arthritis and colitis into the definition of environmental illness.[3,9,20,21]

Thus environmental illness cannot be defined as a disease by using clinical criteria. It is a history of environmental exposure—or presumed exposure—rather than any clinical manifestation that is the basis for diagnosis. Case-finding is impossible unless one uses exposure to define disease. It follows then that environmental illness is not a disease or syndrome, but rather it is a belief that illness *must* be present if an environmental exposure has occurred. This approach to diagnosis leads to a situation in which any possible component of air, food, and water in any amount and in any duration of contact can cause any disease or incite any symptom.

PATHOLOGY

A search of the clinical ecology literature for examples of gross or microscopic tissue pathology specific to environmental illness is totally unrewarding.

THEORIES OF IMMUNOPATHOGENESIS

Clinical ecology theories encompass elements of immunologic hypersensitivity, immune complex pathology, autoimmunity, and defective regulation of the immune response. Often a combination of these mechanisms is used to explain both etiology of disease and production of symptoms in established disease.

The term "chemical hypersensitivity syndrome" implies allergy, but clinical ecologists do not believe that the release of mast cell mediators by IgE antibodies is responsible for environmental illness in their patients. Some claim that abnormally low serum levels of IgE are characteristic of environmental illness, but examination of their data does not show this to be the case. Although several of their studies claim that inflammatory mediators of immediate hypersensitivity are abnormal and further altered by chemical exposure, these studies lack sufficient controls to be conclusive. Reported symptoms bear no similarity to any of the well-defined IgE mediated diseases.

An immune complex etiology is based on reports of circulating immune complexes and altered serum concentrations of complement components. However, the "abnormalities" in these reports are probably consistent with normal variations found in a healthy adult population.[33] Immune complex deposition has not been shown by the usual immunoflourescence techniques, and evidence of vasculitis clinically or pathologically has never been demonstrated in patients with environmental illness. The occasional references to a possible autoimmune mechanism in the clinical ecology literature are not supported by a consistent clinical history, by the presence of circulating autoantibodies, or by evidence of tissue-specific inflammation consistent with an autoimmune pathogenesis.

Theories based on hypersensitivity, immune complex disease, and autoimmunity would predict that clinical ecology patients have antibodies to the environmental chemicals and foods believed to cause disease in each case. Sensitive and specific testing methods for detecting and quantitating antibodies in serum and other body fluids are readily available, but these are not used by clinical ecologists. They opt instead for the method of symptom provocation. This procedure has never been shown to detect—or even correlate with—any type of immune response. Neutralization (i.e., elimination) of symptoms by minute amounts of chemicals or other substances given by injection or absorbed sublingually has likewise never been shown to eliminate antibodies or immune complexes.

Theories based on toxic damage to T lymphocytes by environmental chemicals are currently in vogue among clinical ecologists. They contend that almost any chemical or food can damage the immune system by disturbing a "normal" helper-to-suppressor T lymphocyte ratio, thereby causing either deficient or excessive antibody production by B lymphocytes. There is in fact no experimental or clinical evidence to show that abnormal circulating levels of any lymphocyte subsets characterize these patients. Helper-to-suppressor T cell ratios normally vary over a wide range,[14] and there is no reason to interpret the ratio *per se* as a pathogenic factor. There is no experimental support for the statement that suppressor T cells are more susceptible to damage by environmental chemicals than are helper T cells, and the range of chemicals cited as disease-causing by clinical ecologists is so wide and heterogeneous as to make a theory based on a uniform toxic effect highly implausible.

Clinical ecologists use certain concepts that are outside the realm of current immunologic knowledge. "Masked food sensitivity," "spreading phenomenon" and "chemical overload" are concepts used by clinical ecologists to explain the appearance or disappearance of symptoms under certain conditions of diet and chemical exposure. Masked food sensitivity refers to the appearance of symptoms when a food is eaten after having removed it from the diet for several days and the subsequent disappearance of symptoms when the same food is eaten daily. The phenomenon cannot be explained immunologically using either an allergenic or immunotoxic model. Furthermore, the phenomena itself has never been subjected to a placebo-controlled double-blind method of analysis to prove its existence. Clinical ecologists use the term "spreading phenomenon" for the idea that exposure to a particular environmental substance leads to the induction of additional new environmental sensitivities to other (noncross-reacting) substances. In fact, immune responses to different antigens are generally independent events, at least at the level of natural exposure to environmental antigens. Finally, the "chemical overload" concept seems to be borrowed from the phenomenon of reticuloendothelial blockade. As used by clinical ecologists, however, overload concept appears simply to explain the appearance of symptoms at a particular level of presumed exposure to one or more environmental substances.

LABORATORY EVIDENCE OF IMMUNOPATHOLOGY.

As discussed above, a review of the laboratory data obtained from patients with environmental illness as presented in the clinical ecology literature fails to support the concept of an immunologic illness. An independent analysis of 50 cases of environmental illness seen for a second opinion showed that circulating levels of immunoglobulins, complement components, and lymphocyte subsets were normally distributed in most cases, the exceptions being several patients with elevated IgA and B cell counts related to a prior history of respiratory or cutaneous infection.[32]

THE PROVOCATION-NEUTRALIZATION TESTING METHODOLOGY.

The procedure most often used by clinical ecologists for diagnosing multiple chemical and food sensitivities was described in detail so that the reader can appreciate the subjective nature of the test and the ease with which suggestion can influence the patient's response. The procedure has been the subject of a number of published reports; those claiming diagnostic effectiveness are inadequately controlled, whereas those investigations employing adequate controls clearly demonstrate that active and placebo extracts are indistinguishable under the conditions used in clinical ecology practice.[1,10,11] A report that sublingual provocation with food and chemical extracts produced more symptoms than placebo under double-blind conditions is not definitive because distilled water was used as "placebo" and therefore could have been detected in the mouth by taste and texture as distinguished from concentrated protein extracts in glycerinated saline.[12]

THE "DISEASE" COURSE AND ITS RESPONSE TO CLINICAL ECOLOGY TREATMENT

Although clinical ecologists are convinced that their methods of diagnosis can detect an environmentally-caused immunologic disease and that their therapeutic efforts are successful in alleviating symptoms, they have not published any reports describing the natural course of the disease nor its response to treatment. A review of cases examined from 3 months to 6½ years (mean of 2 years) following the clinical ecology diagnosis of environmental illness and the initiation of avoidance and neutralization therapy revealed that only two patients improved as assessed by the number and severity of symptoms. More than half of the patients (26 of 50) were symptomatically worse, and the remainder unchanged.[32] The persistence of symptoms, worsening of symptoms, and appearance of additional new symptoms during therapy attest to a pattern of fear of the everyday environmental engendered by an unfounded perception of an environmentally-damaged immune system.

SUMMARY

The concept of multiple chemical hypersensitivities as a disease entity in which the patient experiences numerous symptoms from numerous chemicals and foods caused by a disturbance of the immune systems lacks a scientific foundation. Published reports of such cases are anecdotal and without proper controls. There is no convincing evidence for any immunologic abnormality in these cases. Diagnostic methods have been shown to be unreliable. Diagnosis, treatment, and theoretical concepts underlying the purported disease are not consistent with current immunologic knowledge and theory. As defined and presented by its proponents, multiple chemical hypersensitivities constitutes a belief and not a disease.

REFERENCES

1. American Academy of Allergy: Position statements: controversial techniques. J Allergy Clin Immunol 67:333, 1981.
2. American Academy of Allergy and Immunology: Position statement: clinical ecology. J Allergy Clin Immunol 78:269, 1986.
3. Bell IR: Clinical Ecology. Bolinas, CA, Common Knowledge Press, 1982.
4. California Medical Association Scientific Board Task Force on Chemical Ecology: Clinical ecology—a critical appraisal. West J Med 144:239, 1986.
5. Committee on Environmental Hypersensitivities: Report of the Ad Hoc Committee on Environmental Hypersensitivity Disorders. Toronto, Ont., Ministry of Health, 1985, p 228.
6. Crayton JW, Stone T, Stein G: Epilepsy precipitated by food sensitivity; report of a case with double-blind placebo-controlled assessment. Clin Encephalog 12:192, 1981.
7. Crook WG: the Yeast Connection; a Medical Breakthrough, 2nd ed. Jackson, TN, Professional Books, 1984.
8. Dickey LD: Clinical genitourinary allergy. Cutis 15:854, 1975.
9. Dickey LD: Clinical Ecology. Springfield, IL, Charles C Thomas Publisher, 1976, p 90.
10. Golbert TM: A review of controversial diagnostic and therapeutic techniques employed in allergy. J Allergy Clin Immunol 56:170, 1975.
11. Jewett DL, Greenberg MR: Placebo responses in intradermal provocation testing with food extracts. J Allergy Clin Immunol 75:205, 1985 (abstract).
12. King DS: Can allergic exposure provoke psychological symptoms? A double-blind test. Biol Psychiatry 16:3, 1981.
13. Levine SA, Reinhardt JH: Biochemical-pathology initiated by free radicals, oxidant chemicals,

and therapeutic drugs in the etiology of chemical hypersensitivity disease. Orthomol Psychiatry 12:166, 1983.

14. Lifson JO, Finch SL, Sasaki DT, Engleman EG: Variables affecting T-lymphocyte subsets in a volunteer blood donor population. Clin Immunol Immunopathol 36:151, 1986.

15. McGovern JJ, Lazaroni JA, Hicks MF, et al: Food and chemical sensitivity. Arch Otolaryngol 109:292, 1983.

16. McGovern JJ, Lazaroni JA, Saifer P, et al: Clinical evaluation of the major plasma and cellular measures of immunity. Orthomol Psychiatry 12:60, 1983.

17. Randolph TG: Allergic-type reactions to industrial solvents and liquid fuels; mosquito abaterment fogs and mists; motor exhausts; indoor utility gas and oil fumes; chemical additives of foods and drugs; and synthetic drugs and cosmetics. J Lab Clin Med 44:910, 1954.

18. Randolph TG: Depressions caused by home exposure to gas and cumbustion products of gas, oil, and coal. J Lab clin Med 46:942, 1955.

19. Randolph TG: The specific adaptation syndrome. J Lab Clin Med 48:934, 1956.

20. Randolph TG: Human Ecology and Susceptibility to the Chemical Environment. Springfield, IL, Charles C Thomas Publisher, 1962.

21. Randolph TG, Moss RW: An Alternative Approach to Allergies. New York, Lippincott and Cromwell, 1980.

22. Rea WJ: Environmentally triggered thrombophlebitis. Ann Allergy 37:101, 1976.

23. Rea WJ: Environmentally triggered small vessel vasculitis. Ann Allergy 38:245, 1977.

24. Rea WJ, Peters DW, Smiley RE, et al: Recurrent environmentally triggered thrombophlebitis: a five-year follow-up. Ann Allergy 38:245, 1977.

25. Rea WJ: Environmentally triggered cardiac disease. Ann Allergy 40:243, 1978.

26. Rea WJ, Bell IR, Suits CW, Smiley RW: Food and chemical susceptibility after environmental chemical overexposure; case histories. Ann Allergy 41:101, 1978.

27. Rinkel HJ, Randolph TG, Zeller M: Food Allergy. Springfield, IL, Charles C Thomas, 1950.

28. Rinkel HJ: The management of food allergy. IV. Food and mold allergy. Arch Otolaryngol 77:302, 1963.

29. Rowe AH: Clinical Allergy. Philadelphia, Lea and Febiger, 1937.

30. Selye H: The general adaptation syndrome and the diseases of adaptation. J Allergy 17:231, 1946.

31. Speer F: The allergic tension-fatigue syndrome. Pediatr Clin N Amer 1:1029, 1954.

32. Terr AI: Environmental illness: a clinical review of 50 cases. Arch Intern Med 146:145, 1986.

33. Toth CA, Phol D, Aguello V: Methods for detection of immune complexes by utilizing C1q or rheumatoid factors. *In* Rose NR, Friedman H, Fahey JL (eds): Manual of Clinical Laboratory Immunology, 3rd ed. Washington, American Society for Microbiology, 1986, pp 204–210.

CARROLL M. BRODSKY, PhD, MD

MULTIPLE CHEMICAL SENSITIVITIES AND OTHER "ENVIRONMENTAL ILLNESS": A PSYCHIATRIST'S VIEW

This paper concerns itself with a treatment philosophy and approach called clinical ecology, with the physicians who utilize it, and with the patients treated by it, and with the network of reactions engendered by Clinical Ecology and those who oppose it. It is based on a study of "allergic-to-everything" patients described in an earlier report.[5] Since that time the subject has provoked a substantial body of literature and many more such patients have been studied. The controversy continues — are these patients sick or well, are their symptoms physical or mental, are they disabled from work, and do they need to live in special environments?

In all cultures, social norms determine definitions of "health" and "illness," and the expected role behavior of both those regarded as "sick" and their "healers." Western industrial societies view illness primarily as a malfunctioning of the body, including the brain, to be corrected by socially-approved and appropriate medical and surgical interventions. "Modern" medicine has also tended to separate mental from physical illness, with doctors concentrating on diagnosing physical "disease" in patients presenting with bodily complaints and on administering effective treatments.[22] If the patients experience relief of symptoms, both they and their physicians are satisfied and their role behaviors have been reinforced — the patient has gotten "well" and the doctor has "healed."

Some members of our society experience chronic bodily symptoms for which there appears to be no adequate physical explanation.[8,29,30,34,36] Despite an often substantial period of searching, entailing diverse treatments from multiple physicians, these individuals are unable to find doctors who can provide an acceptable, consistent, and coherent diagnosis and who can institute lasting helpful treatment. Many of these patients shift from one specialist to another, going from family physicians to allergists to neurologists and other medical specialists, and to chiropractors, acupuncturists, homeopaths, and even faith healers. Both the patients and their physicians feel frustrated and dissatisfied, the patients because they remain convinced that their symptoms signal a physical disorder for which a medical explanation must exist and the physicians because they have been impotent as healers, unable to help these obviously distressed individuals or to reassure them that they do not have a serious disease. Such patients are time-consuming and in clinic settings not infrequently are objects of derision.[2,19,45]

From the Department of Psychiatry, University of California, San Francisco, School of Medicine, San Francisco, California

Reprint requests to Carroll M. Brodsky, PhD, MD, Department of Psychiatry, University of California, San Francisco, School of Medicine, San Francisco, California 94143

Many physicians reject such patients immediately after taking a history and examining them, recognizing that they do not have the tools for treating such people. Other physicians take on such patients, recognizing that, although there is no "treatment" available for them, these patients do need support and care and protection from physicians who might prescribe radical and potentially harmful treatments, in spite of the fact that there is no scientific basis for such prescription.

This paper describes a medical subculture composed of a group of such patients who have found a group of physicians, clinical ecologists, who believe that their treatments can help these patients. The diagnostic and therapeutic treatment methods of these physicians are not considered scientific by the medical establishment and by the specialty groups who would ordinarily review and authorize such treatments, and insurance companies and government agencies have generally resisted paying for such treatment.[7,10,21,31,32,49] Private and public agencies that provide disability benefits argue that these patients are not truly disabled, although those dealing with them recognize that they are in great distress.[11,12]

A review of medical history and literature that reflects on medical cultures reveals that there have always been people who have had unpleasant physical and emotional symptoms and experiences for which they sought explanations.[15,24,26] The explanations ranged from supernatural to preternatural to frankly magical explanations.[50] Running parallel to all of these were biological or medical explanations.[13,43] During most eras of recorded history, explanations from these sources coexisted, varying only in the degree to which one or another predominated for an era or for a subcultural group.[28]

Cultural determinants for evaluating these various components of the treatment of physical and mental symptoms have shifted in the direction of "science."[22] The rise of what is called the scientific method has tended to reassure physicians that they can say "There is nothing wrong with you" and "You don't have a known disease." When they say, "I don't know what is wrong with you," they frequently mean, "I don't believe there is anything wrong with you." When they say, "I can't help you," they frequently mean, "Not only can I not help you, but I don't believe that anyone else can help you."[18]

From time to time physicians, either individually or as a group, challenge the medical scientific establishment of their era, proclaiming that they have physical explanations and physical treatments for conditions that other physicians explain as being purely functional or subjective or psychological.[25] Physicians who categorize themselves under the rubric of clinical ecology are such a group of physicians and have formed a recognizable medical society and subculture that is at odds with the existing western health care establishment.[3,17,20,23,37,41] Parsons and Shils[35] define a "subculture" as a system of beliefs, ideas, and values shared by a subdivision of a cultural unit, certain aspects of which distinguish that subdivision from the larger social group. The shared patterns of orientation and shared frames of reference define, unify, and maintain this subsystem. One factor noted to be key to the persistence is the "reinforcement of group consciousness experienced in political struggles."[25]

For more than 20 years, clinical ecologists have unsuccessfully sought recognition and acceptance from mainstream medicine and regulatory agencies. They continue to exist on the medical periphery, having formed their own formal association with its own official journal. They fill a medical need in that they attract a group of difficult patients who, by and large, are not deemed treatable by traditional practitioners. By legitimating these patients' complaints and by offering definitive treatment in the face of continuing "scientific" opposition, they have restored hope to their patients, who now join and support clinical ecologists in their struggle for official recognition.

WHAT IS CLINICAL ECOLOGY?

The specialty of clinical ecology is described in the preface of each issue of its journal *Clinical Ecology*, as "an orientation in medical practice dedicated to maintenance of health by recognition, management, and prevention of ecologic illness." The definition goes on to explain that "clinical" coupled with "ecology" means "pertaining to or founded on actual observation and treatment of patients, as distinguished from theoretical or basic sciences, in the branch of biology that deals with mutual relationships between organisms and there environments." Ecologic illness is "usually a polysymptomatic, multisystem chronic disorder manifested by adverse relations to environmental excitants, as they are modified by individual susceptibility in terms of specific adaptation." These excitants are present in "air, water, food, drugs, and out habitat."

One of the emphases that distinguishes clinical ecology in practice from other areas of environmental medicine is that the onset of illness depends on the total stress load, including all of the psychosocial, physical, chemical, antigenic, and infective stressors that impinge on the individual. Low doses of substances that singly might be benign may interact additively or synergistically on some common pathways in the body to produce illness.[3]

Recognition of ecologic disorders is by an ecologically-oriented medical history and "objective" physical examination. Ecologic diagnostic procedures are based on observing a patient's response to "re-exposure to a suspected excitant after a period of complete avoidance. When a state of nonadaptation has been achieved by a proper period of avoidance, re-exposure to a common food or potentially toxic environmental chemical can produce a diagnostically significant response." Both management and prevention are effected by "environmental control of identified or suspected excitant exposures; dietary manipulation by a rotary diversified diet of compatible, food and water that is chemically less contaminated; and nutritional supplementation when indicated." Unavoidable reactions to specific identified environmental excitants can often be controlled by "optimal dose immunotherapy" in the presence of active symptoms that is administered either intracutaneously or sublingually. "Symptom-suppressive pharmacological therapy" is seldom necessary. The non-invasive concepts and techniques of clinical ecology, the preface notes, are applicable in the practice of any physician who is directly involved in patient care.

THE PHILOSOPHIC BASIS OF CLINICAL ECOLOGY

The Society of Clinical Ecology was founded in 1965 and was renamed the American Academy of Environmental Medicine in 1985.[39,41] From the beginning it was powered by a "growing dissatisfaction with the national allergy societies as forums for new and broader ideas." These societies, clinical ecologists believed, were departing from the original broad concept of allergy as altered reactions and were restricting the concept narrowly to those conditions mediated by known immunological mechanisms. This eliminated common foods and environmental chemicals from serious consideration until an immunological mechanism could be demonstrated, recognized, and accepted.

In contrast, clinical ecology "is interested in the interactions between the individual man and this constant intake and immediate surroundings, as these may be demonstrated to be reflected in his total health."[17] It was equally concerned with the "relatively new chemical environment." In Randolph's view,[38] the field of allergy has taken two main and "progressively polarized courses" — endogeny, or traditional allergy with its anthropocentric emphasis, and exogeny, which is environmentally focused. "The upshot of these developments," Randolph continues, has been the "increasing tendency to treat both infections and allergic processes by means of drugs aimed to alleviate symptoms or to alter the bodily mechanisms involved (endogeny), rather than to identify, minimize, or neutralize the impingement of specific environmental exposures (exogeny)."[38] This points up one of the major philosophical differences between clinical ecology and traditional allergy, i.e., that clinical ecology considers the environment to be sick and the subject for study and believes that the patient would be well absent the noxious outside factors.[44] Clinical ecology is concerned with "exogenous excitants of chronic illness" that if not identified or controlled are regarded to be safe and allowed to proliferate. Synthetic drugs, chemical pollutants, and systemic yeast infections are examples of agents to which "extreme degrees of individual susceptibility are capable of developing."[38] The results of "environmental excitants of symptom responses" can be the more advanced systemic manifestations of mental and behavioral syndromes, sometimes mediated by "immune dysregulation," which patients have either had all of their lives or which they have acquired as a result of insult to their immune system by toxic substances in the environment.[40] Clinical ecologists seldom indicate to a patient that there is nothing wrong and that the symptoms are entirely subjective and unrelated to biologic etiologies. Instead, they tend to believe that where there is smoke, there is fire, where there are symptoms, there is physical disease.

The manifestations of clinical ecologic illness are protean and are divided by Randolph into localized and systemic syndromes,[40] which commonly are developed from individual susceptibilities, although they may be related to or complicated by infection or hormonal or other influences. *Localized* manifestations include respiratory (rhinitis, bronchitis, asthma, eye and ear syndromes), dermatologic (pruritus, eczema, hives), gastrointestinal (stomatitis, esophagitis, gastritis, colitis, pruritus ani), and genitourinary (urgency, frequency). *Systemic* manifestation include cardiovascular (edema, vasculitis, arrhythmia, hypertension, purpura), rheumatic (arthralgia, arthritis, myalgia, "growing pains") neurologic (fatigue, headache, seizures), and "mental behavioral" ("brain fag," depression, stupor).

THE PATIENTS AND THE EXPLANATIONS

The experience of most of the physicians who have studied clinical ecology patients has been that these patients are intelligent and frequently sophisticated in their understanding of biology and medicine. Not uncommonly, these patients have been trained in and/or have worked in the chemical industry or in medical or paramedical specialities or may be relatives of such persons. Many of the physicians who concentrate in the field of clinical ecology suffered similar complaints or have had family members who were afflicted or may themselves have been treated by clinical ecologists and thus accepted as valid the explanations of clinical ecology. Such patients require more sophisticated explanations for their symptoms than are provided by, for example, chiropractic medicine.

The theories of chiropractic medicine were probably more readily accepted as explanations in an era before citizens became so acutely aware of the potential health and life-threatening dangers in the environment, dangers that they often cannot see and that affect physiologic systems rather than anatomic structures.[1,6,33] Society has become frighteningly aware that chemicals and radiation can produce damage, the results of which are not manifested for years. People have learned that environmental substances can cause ills ranging from cancer to impotence to birth defects to sudden death.[46,47] Individuals who are especially health conscious or body-focused and who experience symptoms will look for explanations and treatments, the elements of which being at least somewhat compatible with culturally-recognized diseases and their accepted causes.

In the culture of 20th century medicine, a disorder of the immune system would represent a sophisticated and acceptable explanation, because the immune system is demonstrably complex and is interrelated with all other systems, and no one would disagree that many of its mechanisms and manifestations are still unknown. Therefore, environmental causes of immune system disorders could explain many human illnesses, including psychiatric syndromes.[42,48]

Clinical ecology explanations also tap into cultural, medical and lay concepts of the health hazards of toxic chemicals and of allergies to food and other ingested substances.[14] We know that allergic reactions may be delayed following exposure and may affect multiple systems of the body. This, too, lends public credence to the theories of clinical ecologists.

THE FOCUS ON CLINICAL ECOLOGY

It is not surprising that clinical ecology is a theory and treatment method that has become a focus of current interest among members of the medical profession and among others who are involved in providing health care. The public, the news media, government agencies, and medical organizations are involved in reviewing the tenets and the results of treatment of clinical ecology. For some, clinical ecology arouses interest, study, and enthusiasm because it challenges a medical establishment that proclaims itself authoritative in research and in determining the standards of practice. Clinical ecology rejects some of the findings, methods and logic of the medical establishment, or at least states that the medical establishment has not come to the right conclusions about its own findings. Clinical ecologists disagree with the observations and laboratory results of physicians who are not adherents of clinical ecology. Frequently the results found in the laboratories of clinical ecologists are different from those found in university laboratories.

Those medical groups that do not accept clinical ecology react to it far more intensely than they do to nonphysician alternative health care approaches.[10,21] Clinical ecologists are physicians, are graduates of the same medical schools, and frequently have gone through the same specialty training programs as have those who oppose them. Not challenging them would suggest that the medical establishment accepts their views. The medical establishment must challenge the views of medical physicians that run counter to what it sees as scientifically proven explanations and practices.[25]

I believe that most of those involved in the controversy, both clinical ecologists and nonclinical ecologists, would agree that the following represent major elements of the evolution of clinical ecology:

- Clinical ecology can be understood as one manifestation of a paradigm in which a theory and set of practices are established to explain the cause of a mental or physical disorder and to prescribe for the treatment of such disorders.
- Patients not helped by previous treatments are referred to practitioners of this new approach, in part because no one else has helped them. Some patients find that they are aided by this approach and they are grateful. They refer more patients. Other physicians are impressed by the theory and what seems to be the success of treatment and join their fellow physicians.

Most physicians do not accept the theory of the treatment of clinical ecology and most patients do not accept the theory of the treatment. Controversy results.

Those who believe become defensive and aggressive. Those who do not believe become more aggressive.

Clinical ecologists claim that research is being done and the results are on the way.[4] So far they have produced little that convinces academic allergists and immunologists that clinical ecology has any merit. Each side accuses the other of bias and unscientific research. Although a few shift positions, for the most part, each group of patients and physicians remains intact. An impasse is reached. The matter is argued before medical associations and ultimately in the courts, which must decide if the patient has a condition that entitles him to treatment and that disables him from work.[16] Those who agree with a given judicial decision cite it as proof of their scientific position.

A SUBJECT FOR STUDY

From the standpoint of medical anthropology, clinical ecology represents an opportunity to study an evolving medical social group and an evolving medical subculture. The medical anthropologist can study the professionals, the leaders, the priestly members of the society, as well as those who approach it to be admitted, those who go through the rites of passages, those who are accepted or rejected. We can understand the elements that support the system and those that undermine it. We can study the society and the subculture and their evolution.

Clinical ecology has meaning for the medical establishment itself. It tells the medical establishment that patients from whom it cannot provide will trigger the development of an alternative health care system such as clinical ecology, a system that has come into being at least in part because there were patients who were dissatisfied with what the medical establishment had to offer. Clinical ecology also informs traditional practitioners that such patients will join alternative health care providers to form not only a medical entity but a political constituency.

Clinical ecology raises the question of who controls treatment practices, who controls treatment standards, and whether patients have a right to be treated in the way in which they want to be treated, even if that treatment is considered ineffective or harmful by the medical establishment. Further, it raises the question of whether these patients have the right to expect others to pay for such medical treatment.

When one looks at clinical ecology itself and its patients, one sees a beleaguered group, the physician members of which feel misunderstood and rejected by their colleagues, while the patients in this group feel unsupported by most physicians, by insurance companies, and sometimes by their families and society generally. Because most physicians are not adherents of the belief system of clinical ecology, the patient has very few physicians to whom to turn when in crisis or in doubt.

The medical establishment finds itself in a bind vis-a-vis the kinds of patients who go to clinical ecologists. Medicine has been accused of overtreating or treating nonspecifically or prolonging treatment without indications for its interventions. Therefore, medicine is understandably reluctant to continue to schedule visits for and treating patients for whom it has no specific treatments.

RECOMMENDATIONS

Long ago, psychiatry recognized that it had no treatments that would resolve the problems and symptoms of many of its patients, but that these sometimes desperate patients needed human contact, advice, an opportunity to ventilate, and reassurance. It described its interventions with such patients as "supportive" psychotherapy.[9,27]

Other physicians must provide supportive treatment for certain patients. Such treatment would consist of acknowledging that the patient's symptoms are very real and very frightening for the patient. In order to reassure he patient, thorough physical examination and laboratory studies should be conducted, sometimes more frequently than is indicated by objective signs. Just as a physician might repeat an electrocardiogram on a patient who has a cardiac fixation or neurosis, so, too, one might need to do repeat tests with the patients described in this report.

The physician should discuss the results of testing with the patient in great detail. Similarly, the physician should repeatedly discuss the hazards of a treatment that is not in response to objective findings or to a pattern of symptoms that are pathognomonic of a disease. The patient should be informed of the harm that such treatment might do and how it might confuse the diagnostic picture. The patient should be told what is the truth, namely, that the physician's approach is a rational one designed to protect the patient.

The physician should accept the patient's condition as chronic and should help the patient accept that. The physician should not suggest that the patient can will away the symptoms. The physician should discourage avoidances that limit the patient's social functioning, but should also recognize that some of the avoidances have the qualities of phobic responses and therefore should not press the patient to be counterphobic.

Physicians taking this approach will not solve the problems of those who would otherwise enter the clinical ecology subculture, but the absence of this approach will leave more people seeking responsive treatment.

SUMMARY

The clinical ecology subculture, like earlier medical subcultures, is the product of patient concerns that the medical establishment cannot allay by treatment or by reassurance. For social and behavioral scientists, it represents a "natural" experiment that can be studied. For those physicians who believe that clinical ecology is without scientific basis generally and/or that its practitioners interpret laboratory results incorrectly, it is a challenge and an irritant. The clinical ecologist-physician feels rejected and the victim of bias and unfair attack. The patient in this subculture feels that finally he has found someone who understands him and is trying to help him, but that he must pay the price of being disapproved or rejected by his former physicians.

REFERENCES

1. Bardana EJ Jr: Office epidemics. Why are Americans suddenly allergic to the workplace? The Sciences 26:39–44, 1986.
2. Barsky AJ, Klerman GL: Overview: hypochondriasis, bodily complaints, and somatic styles. Am J Psychiat 140:273–283, 1983.
3. Bell IR: Clinical Ecology: A New Medical Approach to Environmental Illness. Bolinas, California, Common Knowledge Press, 1982.

4.   Bell IR, King DS: Psychological and physiological research relevant to clinical ecology: overview of current literature. Clin Ecol 1:15–25, 1982.

5.   Brodsky CM: "Allergic to everything": a medical subculture. Psychosomatics 24:731–742, 1983.

6.   Brodsky CM: Psychological factors contributing to somatoform diseases attributed to the workplace. The case of intoxication. J Occup Med 25:459–464, 1983.

7.   Brody JE: Clinical ecology: uncertain quantity. The New York Times, 1/2/85, pp. 11–12.

8.   Brown HN, Vaillant GE: Hypochondriasis. Arch Intern Med 1412:723–726, 1981.

9.   Buckley P: Supportive psychotherapy — a neglected treatment. Psychiat Ann 16:515–521, 1986.

10. California Medical Association Scientific Board Task Force on Clinical Ecology: Clinical ecology — a critical appraisal. West J Med 144:239–245, 1986.

11. Canadian Ministry of Health, Ontario: Report of the Ad Hoc Committee on Environmental Hypersensitivity Disorders, August, 1985, appendices.

12. Canadian Ministry of Health, Ontario: Report on the Advisory Panel on Environmental Hypersensitivity, September, 1986.

13. Carter KC: Germ theory, hysteria, and Freud's early work in psychopathology. Med Hist 24:259–274, 1980.

14. Check W: Eat, drink, and be merry — or argue about food "allergy." JAMA 250:701–711, 1983.

15. Cheyne G: The English Malady: On a Treatise of Nervous Diseases of All Kinds, as Spleen, Vapors, Lowness of Spirits, Hypochondriasis, and Hysterical Distempers. London, 1733, p. 11, *Cited in* Kellner R: Somatization and Hypochondriasis. New York, Praeger Scientific, 1986, p. 3.

16. Davis ES: The legal side of ecological illness. Clin Ecol 4:77–80, 1986.

17. Dickey LK (ed): Clinical Ecology. Springfield, IL, Charles C Thomas Press, 1976.

18. Drossman DA: The problem patient. Evaluation and care of medical patients with psychosocial disturbances. Ann Intern Med 88:366–372, 1978.

19. Earley LW, Von Mering O: Growing old the outpatient way. Am J Psychiat 125:135–139, 1969.

20. Editorial: Hypersensitive. San Francisco Chronicle, p. 15, August 6, 1984.

21. Executive Committee of the American Academy of Allergy: Position statement-controversial techniques. J Allergy Clin Immunol 67:333–338, 1981.

22. Fabrega H Jr: The idea of medicalization: an anthropological perspective. Perspectives Biol Med 24:129–142, 1980.

23. Finston P: Environmental "cerebral allergies" . . . fact of fad? The Psychiatric Times, March, 1986, pp. 4–6 passim.

24. Fischer-Homberger E: Hypochondriasis of the eighteenth century - neurosis of the present century. Bull Hist Med 46:391–401, 1972.

25. Goode WJ: Encroachment, charlatanism, and the emerging profession: psychology, sociology, and medicine. Am Soc Rev 25:902–914, 1960.

26. Gosling FS: Neurasthenia in Pennsylvania: a perspective on the origins of American psychotherapy, 1870–1910. J Hist Med Allied Sci 40:188–206, 1985.

27. Karasu TB: Supportive psychotherapy. Psychosomatic medicine and psychotherapy. Psychiat Ann 16:522–525, 1986.

28. Kaufman M: Homeopathy in America. The Rise and Fall of a Medical Heresy. Baltimore, The Johns Hopkins Press, 1971.

29. Kellner R: Hypochondriasis and atypical somatoform disorder. *In* Greist JH, Jefferson JW, Spitzer RL (eds.) Treatment of Mental Disorders. New York, Oxford University Press, 1982, pp. 286–303.

30. Kellner R Somatization and Hypochondriasis. New York, Praeger Scientific, 1986.

31. Marshall E: Immune system theories on trial. Science 234:1490–1492, 1986.

32. Marshall E: Woburn case may spark explosion of lawsuits. Science 234:418–420, 1986.

33. McGuire R: Can't hide from pollution indoors. Medical Tribune, January 7, 1987, pp. 6 passim.

34. McKenna PJ: Disorders with overvalued ideas. Br J Psychiat 145:579–585, 1984.

35. Parsons T, Shils EA: Toward a General Theory of Action. Cambridge, Harvard University Press, 1951.

36. Quill TE: Somatization disorder. One of medicine's blind spots. JAMA 254:3075–3079, 1985.

37. Raeburn P: Chemical allergy theory discredited. San Jose Mercury News, April 16, 1985, pp. 1E passim.

38. Randolph TG: The development of ecologically focused medical care. Clin Ecol 3:6–16, 1985.

39. Randolph TG: Emergence of the specialty of clinical ecology. Clin Ecol 1:84–90, 1982–83.

40. Randolph TG: Graphic representation of clinical ecology. Clin Ecol 2:27–33, 1983.
41. Randolph TG: Historical development of clinical ecology. *In* Dickey LD (ed): Clinical Ecology. Springfield, IL: Charles C Thomas, 1976, pp. 9–17.
42. Rogers MP, Dubey D, Reich P: The influence of the psyche and the brain on immunity and disease susceptibility: a critical review. Psychosom Med 41:147–164, 1979.
43. Rosenberg CE: George M Beard and American nervousness. *In* Rosenberg CE: No Other Gods. On Science and American Social Thought. Baltimore, Johns Hopkins University Press, 1976, pp. 98–108.
44. Randolph TG, Moss RW: Allergies: Your Hidden Enemy. How the new science of clinical ecology is unravelling the causes of mental and physical illness. Wellingborough (Canada), Turnstone Press, 1981.
45. Smith GR, Monson RA, Ray DC: Patients with multiple unexplained symptoms. Their characteristics, functional health, and health care utilization. Arch Intern Med 146:69–72, 1986.
46. Smith HM: The ultimate allergy—to the 20th century. MD July, 1983, pp. 71–81.
48. Stein M, Schiavi RC, Camerino M: Influence of brain and behavior on the immune system. Science 191:435–440, 1976.
47. Spake A: Medical nightmare — a new American nightmare? MS March, 1986, 35–42 passim.
49. Terr AI: Environmental illness: a clinical review of 50 cases. Arch Intern Med 146:145–149, 1986.
50. Tuan Y-F: Fear of disease. *In* Tuan Y-F: Landscapes of Fear. New York: Pantheon Book, 1979, pp. 87–104.

JUDITH SPARER, MS, CIH

ENVIRONMENTAL EVALUATION OF WORKERS WITH MULTIPLE CHEMICAL SENSITIVITIES: AN INDUSTRIAL HYGIENIST'S VIEW

According to a standard and widely used reference,[1] the charge of traditional industrial hygiene is to protect "nearly all workers." Guidelines are specified "to represent conditions in which it is believed that nearly all workers may be repeatedly exposed day after day without adverse effect." The handbook goes on to say that some workers may experience discomfort at concentrations of some substances below these threshold limit values (TLV's) and even fewer may be affected more seriously because of a pre-existing condition or by development of an occupational illness.

In recent years the issue of the "nearly all workers" has been raised and several articles have been published addressing the question of who those others are and what should or can be done about them.[46] The thrust of these articles is that there are subpopulations whom it is either impossible or impractical to protect but who could be identified, advised of their risk, and either followed until they develop clinical problems or are denied employment in what for them would be a hazardous environment. Although undoubtedly there are many clinical reasons for such individual responses, workers with multiple chemical sensitivities are certainly among those who would fall into that "other" group of reactors at the extreme low end of the dose-response curve.

Because of drastic implications of arbitrarily assigning such workers to an "unprotectable" status, it is crucial that each individual's environment(s) be carefully explored and evaluated to establish where on the appropriate dose/response curve or curves they sit. As I shall try to demonstrate, these patients may be far more protectable than initially imagined if the work-up is performed in the appropriate way and if those who control the environment—usually the employers—are willing to be open-minded and flexible in their interpretation of the results. Premature labeling may obscure documentable environmental disease and lead to complacent acceptance of a work environment that may be hazardous to many more workers than the hypersensitive individual whose extreme symptomatology forces the issue into the open.

To put this in practicable form, I shall begin with a presentation of the basic

Occupational Medicine Program, Department of Internal Medicine, Yale University School of Medicine, New Haven, Connecticut

Reprint requests to Judith Sparer, MS, CIH, Occupational Medicine Program, School of Medicine, 333 Cedar Street, New Haven, CT 06510 approach to the worker environment. Subsequently, some of the subtleties and difficulties will be described by analyzing some of our more challenging cases.

THE GENERAL APPROACH

INFORMATION OBTAINABLE FROM THE PATIENT: HISTORY

It is useful to begin with an occupational history, starting with the current or most recent job and going back as far as possible to get the shape of the person's working life. Find out the job title and something of the working environment at each job. What did the person actually do? Was there any chemical or dust exposure? Did he/she work in an industrial environment or an office environment?

Then focus particular attention on the time period of onset of symptoms. Make sure that you understand what the person's job actually was. What was the function of the place of business (i.e., did thy make widgets or provide legal services?). What products, chemicals, materials were handled and for how much time of the person's time? Was/is there appropriate ventilation? Did any changes at all occur at the workplace? Were new chemicals introduced? New processes or machines? Was any renovation done in the office? New carpeting? Did the trouble arise subsequent to a flood or modification of the ventilation or heating systems? Any change that can be associated with that time period may be a valuable clue. Of course, patients do not always know the answers to all of these questions, and access to information may require some effort on the patient or practitioner's part; general approaches are discussed below.

The same kind of information about non-work environments must be obtained, focusing again on the changes that may have occurred prior to or during the beginning of the illness. Any renovation in the home, pest extermination, or insulation may be important. A move or a change in detergent used, a new hobby practiced or other forms of activity should be noted. Usually the patient should be able to provide these data, though it may require some thought and/or review of household products and practices.

The temporal behavior of the illness may also yield valuable environmental clues. The pattern, if one can be identified, of feeling sometimes better and sometimes worse can point toward specific offending environments. For example, symptoms that emerge during the work week and resolve on weekends—a "better at home and worse at work" story—is helpful. Or, "Since moving to the new house, I haven't been able to breathe!" Care must be taken, though, not to "beg" associations nor to equate automatically temporal with causal relationships.

Patient perception of the "epidemiology" of the problem may also be valuable and should be elicited. Do other people at the workplace have the same problems? If the answer to this question is yes, it is more likely that a common environmental problem, rather than special or unique host factors, is causal. Importantly, such patients may be the key to recognition of "indoor air pollution" or "tight building syndrome" outbreaks. If the patient feels others tolerate his/her environment without symptoms, there may still be an indoor air pollution problem but one that will be more difficult to resolve. One must remember, too, that the complainant may have become so socially isolated by his or her illness that knowledge about the reaction of others has been obscured.

Where possible, the names of specific environmental contaminants should be elicited. Information sheets, called Material Safety Data Sheets (MSDSs), should be available through workplaces and product manufacturers. As of 1986, these MSDSs are required by the Occupational Safety and Health Administration to be available to employees in the manufacturing sector but are now often obtained in the service sector as well. These sheets should identify the toxic components of all materials used in the workplace, giving generic chemical names for ingredients in everything from carpet shampoo to roach spray to widget oil. Without fairly complete information of this sort it is very difficult to pursue the possibility that certain specific exposures may be causing symptoms. Unfortunately, these sheets are not always filled out thoroughly or informatively, i.e., a certain portion of the compound may be listed as "proprietary" or "inert." You may have to call the supplier at the number that should be on the MSDS for more useful information. It will usually be supplied to a physician without objection.

Of course, in order to make sense, this information must be evaluated in the context of the patient's job and practices—how often the chemicals are used, in what proximity to the persons' workstation, etc. Carpet shampooing may be done once a year or once a week. Similarly, a toxic degreasing fluid may be sitting in an open tank on a workbench or may be carefully enclosed and equipped with local exhaust ventilation, a very big difference.

The answers to all these questions provide the basis for subsequent steps, but not always sufficient information to determine whether specific environmental cause(s) can be found to explain symptoms. Occasionally, results of clinical evaluation may be revealing of a specific toxic effect, focusing all further attention on a particular chemical or operation. In patients with complaints of multiple chemical sensitivities, however, this is rarely the case. Usually the environment itself must be investigated further. This is the subject of the next section.

EVALUATION OF THE PATIENT'S ENVIRONMENT

Partly because of tradition, and partly due to the regulatory environment in which we are taught to function, industrial hygienists often tend to approach the environment by first attempting to categorize and to quantify its contaminants. Usually this is done without detailed knowledge of the clinical complaints that may have prompted the investigation nor any epidemiologic information suggesting relationships between the workplace and complaints.

In evaluating the environment of individuals with multiple complaints this approach can be misleading, since it almost invariably leads to the premature conclusion that exposures are "too low" to be causing effects. This circumvents the real issue—whether identifiable or correctable low level exposures may be causing the problem—and may lead the patient and the employer alike into polarized, intransigent views of what is going on. The following case illustrates these problems:

Case 1: We were asked by the administration of a nearby hospital to investigate the case of a supervisor with multiple symptoms that she associated with "the air" in her billing office. Her problems included skin and eye irritation, cough, congestion, and extreme fatigue associated with work. Significantly, other workers in the room also had similar complaints. Steps taken included physical exams for those most affected (which were unrevealing), a "gambit" move of the office to a room down the hall, isolation of old files in a remote room, and the initiation of renovation of the former office space. These changes failed to alleviate the complaints. An environmental consultant was hired to investigate.

The consulting firm sampled air for fiberglass, suspected to be entering the ventilation system from renovation of an adjacent wing of the building. They also sampled for formaldehyde, nuisance dust, ozone, carbon dioxide and organic solvents, "the usual suspects." Carbon dioxide was found to be 600–700 ppm. Others were not found at detectable levels. A general sample of organic solvents revealed only "common solvents at levels significantly below industrial hygiene concern." Later, marked variations by location in organic solvent levels, all well below those levels, were documented by the same consultant.

Based on these results, the employer assumed that no serious environmental hazard existed and attempted to disclaim the problem. Unfortunately, this infuriated the affected employees and symptoms were aggravated. Some months later our group was called for a second opinion.

Consistent with our general approach, we began our work with a simple symptom questionnaire, including an open-ended question to determine what each respondent thought was causing the problem. A second billing office where there were no reported "cases" was used as a control group, allowing us to calculate attack rates and determine that there was a clearly worse than normal situation in the affected department. This epidemiologic fact, as well as the association between symptoms and time spent in the office, was central to our subsequent look at the environment itself. Specific sources of odor or symptoms reported by the patients were also noted. Not unimportantly, we learned that most symptoms had begun only after the onset of a major building renovation.

We next conducted a walk-through of the offices, paying close attention to possible sources of noxious dust or fumes, stressful or harmful work practices and the ventilation. We discovered clear evidence of various construction dusts and fiber throughout the office, several sources of unusual potential contamination, especially carbonless copying forms, and a ventilation system set to recycle office air rather than introduce fresh air. Furthermore, smoking was allowed throughout the area; stale smoke filled the room. Finally, it was apparent that the noise and incovenience of the external renovation was stressors inside the office, as were the impressive numbers of forms.

We concluded that there was an environmental problem, the multi-faceted causes of which included fiberglass and other construction dust, off-gasing from the carbonless copy paper forms, cigarette smoke and lack of fresh air. No further "measurements" were proposed and findings and recommendations were presented to both management and all the employees. Recommendations included clean-up of the fiberglass, air balancing and the provision of increased fresh air to the area and better mixing, the dedication of a separate smoking area, and strong encouragement for the company's plan to drastically reduce the mountains of forms by switching to a computer system. With these recommendations came our assurances that there was no evidence that the present problem would increase the risk of developing disease later on as a result of these exposures.

The follow-up is illuminating. Six months later construction was still going on, the amount of fresh air was claimed to be about 33%–100%, smoking was not permitted, fiberglass and dust were no longer present but the mountains of forms were undiminished. The number of complaints were far fewer but the problems of the index case had become worse. With more experience, we realize that this is not an atypical case. Four years later, complaints continue, fresh air is claimed to be 100% but CO_2 is still twice that of outside air.

As the above case illustrates, potential contaminant sources in the workplace are legion, even in an office, an environment historically considered clean, quiet and free of industrial toxins. An office environment will usually contain a copying machine that may use solvents in copy development or may generate significant amounts of ozone by the high voltages used. Office construction and new furniture may contain particle board emitting formaldehyde; plastics and electronic equipment with trace odors and cleaning compounds may be present. Habitation by people who breathe, work, smoke, and wear perfume in and of itself necessitates some ventilation to minimize irritant effects.

The mechanical ventilation system, in addition to possibly providing inadequate dilution and flushing with fresh air, may be the source or means of distributing the problem. It may be carrying chemicals or flue gases or dust from a remote area or even an outside source and bringing it to an otherwise clean area. It may be lined with fiberglass that is getting into the airstream. It may not be equipped with humidification, resulting in extremely low relative humidity. Less than 40% relative humidity causes severe discomfort to many people. Or it may contain moisture and carry bacteria or molds or other biologically active material into the work areas. Thus, even a seemingly innocuous work environment may be causing illnesses.

Very often environmental data regarding people with MCS will be interpreted out of the context in which they are developed by comparison to applicable OSHA or other industrial standards. In general, in nonindustrial settings pollutants will be identifiable at levels far below these standards. For example, although OSHA currently condones a level of 3 ppm of formaldehyde averaged over 8 hours, never to exceed 10 ppm for more than 30 minutes, levels as low as 0.05 ppm have been associated with persistent respiratory congestion and asthma in some individuals. Formaldehyde is an extremely irritating substance, easily perceived. Other chemicals, too, may cause these typical adverse health effects at levels well below the standards in some susceptible individuals. Consequently, the numbers themselves cannot be readily used to determine whether particular environmental factors may be causal of symptoms. Certainly formaldehyde in almost any quantifiable amount could, for some individuals, be a problem. Other factors are less well studied. Indeed, the effects of complex mixes of traces of many substances have not been studied at all. A lot of money can easily be spent for measurements only to find that nobody knows quite what to make of the results. Day-to-day variation can also be great; at very low levels the range can easily be an order of magnitude or two! Conservatively, the presence of any chemical means it could likely be found at higher levels at other times. Thus, any substance present at levels of 1–10% of established TLVs should be traced to its source and eliminated or managed with local exhaust ventilation, if necessary. The bottom line is, though, that the cost to accurately define the distribution of all contaminants usually far exceeds the benefits. Even if such data could be readily obtained, they often fail to answer the question of causation of the patient's symptoms.

Far more useful than this sort of "fishing in the air" would be a few simpler measures directed toward a solution. Many people are now using carbon dioxide as a marker for the build-up of low-level contaminants. Carbon dioxide is present in the atmosphere at 300–350 ppm and is nontoxic. It is, of course, a by-product of combustion as well as breathing, and is regarded as an asphyxiant gas at 5000 ppm. At 500 ppm in an indoor environment some people report symptoms such as headache and fatigue. At 1500 ppm almost everyone complains. Other symptoms are also reported that may be due to other chemicals present but not measured. In general, any buildup from morning to afternoon is a marker for inadequate ventilation.

LOOKING AT THE VENTILATION

While quantifying levels of particular contaminants is frequently unrewarding, extensive assessment of general and local ventilation is often of major diagnostic and therapeutic importance. Bringing the ventilation system up to standard cures indoor air pollution problems in the vast majority of non-industrial workplaces. A review of the system to make sure it has been properly maintained, that fans are functioning as they should, that fresh air dampers are well placed away from contamination sources and sufficiently open is paramount. Then the amount of fresh air actually being delivered must be calculated. The American Society of Heating, Refrigerating and Air Conditioning Engineers has developed draft guidelines suggesting a minimum of 20 cubic feet per minute (cfm) of fresh air per person, to maintain a CO_2 concentration of less than 1,000 ppm. It has been recommended that new buildings be ventilated with 100% fresh air for the first 6 months and that recirculated air be limited to a maximum of 50% for the next 1–2 years because of off-gasing of modern building materials.[3]

Occasionally cases can be traced to specific causes such as algae in the humidifying system, or mold on a rug that had been flooded during a roof leak, or a carbonless copy paper recently introduced. Most often, a combination of strategies such as reducing sources, providing local exhaust ventilation, providing for better air distribution and mixing, removing mildewed carpet, cleaning heating coils or increasing the fresh air is successful.

To put these findings in perspective, the National Institute for Occupational Safety and Health has reported results of almost 450 non-industrial worksite investigations where one or more worker(s) complained of recurrent symptoms at work; in almost 90% some correctable problem was found[5]:

1. Inadequate ventilation was cited in 52% of the cases. Among the problems were insufficient fresh air supplied, poor distribution and mixing, temperature and humidity extremes or fluctuations, and poor maintenance.

2. Inside contamination, including improperly applied pesticides, boiler additives such as diethylethanolamine, cleaning agents, tobacco smoke, combustion gases and cross-contamination from other locations was the major cause in 17% of the investigations.

3. Outside contamination caused 11% of the problems. This included motor vehicle exhaust, asphalt, solvents, dust and sewer gas that got access to the building through intake plenums, windows, or leaks.

4. Biological contamination was involved in 5% of the investigations. Fungi, bacteria, microbial products and even protozoa can be responsible.

5. In 3% of the cases, building materials such as particle board, fiberglass, glues, adhesives and caulking caused the problem.

THE INDUSTRIAL ENVIRONMENT

The industrial environment presents very different problems to the industrial hygienist. I will illustrate with another case.

Case 2: Mr. G. came to our clinic shortly after recovering from pneumonitis, most likely due to an accidental exposure at work to various irritants, including H_2S and phosphoric acid. As he recovered he noted the onset of respiratory and nervous system complaints to numerous chemicals, both inside and outside the workplace. Although exhaustive medical tests were negative, he was unable to work for over one year. He underwent both group and individual psychotherapy aimed at insight and diminishing symptom amplification; he was also placed on antidepressants for suspected associated depression.

As part of his rehabilitation, the workplace environment was evaluated. Recommendations were made, and because he was a senior and valued employee, modifications to reduce both daily exposures and the risk of accidental over-exposures were made. Mr. G. returned to his original job. Although he continues at the same factory, his work station has been changed and his exposures to chemicals are greatly diminished. Nonetheless, he continues to have recurrent episodes of respiratory distress accompanied by dizziness, but he is permitted fresh air breaks when he feels ill. Lost work time is minimal.

This case illustrates the great value of carefully exploring the environment even when nonenvironmental factors are also clearly important. Although the clinical staff treating Mr. G. suspected the importance of psychological issues subsequent to his accident, definition and manipulation of the work environment played a crucial role in his overall evaluation and treatment. The case also illustrates the importance of "individual" standards and practices for toxins when this is feasible; this patient was able to continue at a skilled job, preventing extreme personal dislocation and likely prolonged illness and disability.

SOLUTIONS

Most professionals are trained in some specific methodology for problem-solving stemming from a universal assumption that the first essential step is to define the problem. In occupational health, when we are unable, as often happens, to make such a definition with satisfactory specificity, one of two things happens: (1) We pour our resources into attempting to elucidate the problem, which is often doomed to failure because of the lack of sufficient knowledge. We keep looking for already identified and "proven" problem causers, which is as yet a severely under-populated category; (2) We define away the problem by concluding that the environmental conditions are "normal" or the incidence rate of illness is "acceptable," hence, no related illness exists. Once we have fallen into either of these two stagnant backwaters, we fail to work to improve conditions by implementing any of the routine measures to improve the environment, and we fail to contribute the understanding of the mechanism of response of those who suffer first and most.

Those affected can be identified with the help of the occupational history discussed earlier. Knowledge of exposure to potential toxins and patterns of illness in coworkers consistent with an environmental source make the likelihood of a correctable problem high. Although the role of specific factors in an individual case may be problematic, with a strong solution-oriented approach, persistance and cooperation, many MCS patients can be, if not completely cured, at least helped.

REFERENCES

1. American Conference of Government and Industrial Hygienists: Threshold Limit, Values and Biological Exposure Indices for 1985–86. Cincinnati, ACGIH, 1985.
2. American Society of Heating, Refrigerating and Air-Conditioning Engineers: Ventilation for Acceptable Indoor Air Quality. Standard (#A62–1981R). July 15, 1986 Public Review Draft. Atlanta, ASHRAE, 1981.
3. Berglund B, Johansson I, Lindvall T: A longitudinal study of air contaminants in a newly build school. Environment International 8:111–5, 1982.
4. DeSilva P: TLVs to protect "nearly all workers." Appl Indus Hyg 1:49–53, 1986.
5. National Institute for Occupational Safety and Health: Guidance for Indoor Air Quality Investigations. Cincinnati, NIOSH, 1987.
6. Lewis TR: Identification of Sensitive Subjects not Adequately Protected by TLVs. Appl Indust Hyg 1:66–9, 1986.

LEO GALLAND, MD

BIOCHEMICAL ABNORMALITIES IN PATIENTS WITH MULTIPLE CHEMICAL SENSITIVITIES

This review presents a retrospective analysis of data gathered on patients with multiple chemical sensitivities (MCS) seen in medical consultation in a non-occupational setting. Control data from a group of allergic patients without clinically apparent chemical or group drug hypersensitivities is presented for comparison. Few studies of this patient population have appeared, and none has included control data. Rea and his colleagues described elevated blood levels of organic pollutants and reduced erythrocyte chromium in MCS.[14,25] Two separate groups failed to find any immunological abnormalities and proposed that "environmental illness" of this type is a psychosomatic illness.[2,31]

Unlike common allergens, the substances to which MCS patients react are inherently toxic and capable of producing neurologic and mucosal damage in anyone at high concentrations.[7] As these substances may produce tissue damage through free-radical formation, among other mechanisms, Levine proposed that MCS represents a failure of anti-oxidant defenses.[15-17] His theory was supported by anecdotal reports of improvement in MCS with the use of anti-oxidants and by the known protective effects of anti-oxidants in ameliorating damage to humans and animals caused by environmental pollutants. His theory influenced the nature of biochemical parameters assessed in the present study.

METHODS

The author maintains a private consultation practice in New York City, which attracts patients with difficult chronic health problems, including many with allergy and MCS. For this report, I selected cases from my office files in which MCS was a presenting primary symptom. I personally reviewed the records of 400 active patients and placed patients in the MCS group if their initial complaints included intolerance of low doses of multiple volatile substances. I excluded a few patients in whom no biochemical assessments relative to the study parameters had been obtained. The control group were patients presenting for treatment of allergy or evaluation of somatic complaints such as fatigue, who denied MCS or drug sensitivity during the initial interview. Patients whose presenting complaints did not include MCS but whose history or clinical course revealed hypersensitivities to numerous drugs and chemicals were excluded.

Reprint requests to Leo Galland, MD, 41 East 60th Street, New York, New York 10022

The following biochemical determinations were obtained, although all were not obtained on each patient:

(1) Serum automated chemistry
(2) Complete blood count
(3) T3, T4, TSH, thyroid antibodies
(4) Serum and erythrocyte mineral levels; magnesium, zinc, copper, and iron
(5) Erythrocyte superoxide dismutase activity[5]
(6) Erythrocyte glutathione peroxidase activity[23]
(7) Blood vitamin levels: A, B_1, B_2, B_3, B_6, C, folic acid, B_{12}, 1,25 dihydroxy vitamin D
(8) Fractionated amino acid excretion
(9) Quantitative fatty acid analysis of serum and phospholipids
(10) Lipid peroxides in blood[33]
(11) Epstein-Barr virus antibodies

Commercial reference laboratories were used for all studies. These included Smith-Kline-Bioscience, Rockland Medi-Labs, Monroe Medical Research Laboratory, and Meridien Clinical Laboratories.

RESULTS

Fifty-six patients met the study criteria for MCS. There were 10 men and 46 women. Ages ranged from 13 to 61 (median 46). All patients complained of multiple hypersensitivities to foods and common inhalant allergens, as well as to environmental chemicals. All were chronically ill, even when avoiding substances to which they reacted. Thirty-six had ceased employment or made major job changes because of their illness.

Mitral valve prolapse had been diagnosed by echocardiography in 11 patients (22%), 10 female and 1 male.

Hypothyroidism was or had been diagnosed in 9 females (20%) and 5 of these had high titres of thyroid antibodies.

Four patients had serological evidence of chronic Epstein-Barr virus infection. Two of them were leukopenic.

Mildly elevated serum transaminase values were present in 5 patients.

The control group consisted of 17 males and 37 females, aged 15 to 60 (mean 48). No patient in this group had ceased work or made a major job change for health reasons.

Mitral valve prolapse was present in 3 females, hypothyroidism in 5 females, and autoimmune thyroiditis in 2.

While female patients are preponderant in both groups, the relative proportion of females is somewhat greater in the MCS group. Females in the MCS group also had a greater frequency of mitral valve prolapse, hypothyroidism and autoimmune thryoiditis. None of the differences reached statistical significance.

Table 1. Nutritional Deficiencies in the MCS and Control Patients

| | | NUMBER DEFICIENT* TOTAL N | |
NUTRIENT	ASSESSMENT	MCS	CONTROL
Vitamin B_6	Serum pyridoxal phosphate	20/32	23/32
Magnesium	Serum	4/54	2/50
	RBC	10/54	10/50
	Urine	3/54	4/50
Vitamin B_{12}	Serum	1/20	1/15
Folic Acid	Serum	5/34	4/20
Zinc	Serum	2/40	5/35
Vitamin C	WBC	5/8	1/3
1,25 Vitamin D	Serum	4/21	1/7
Vitamin B_1	Erythrocyte transketolase	3/17	2/14
Fe	Serum	4/50	2/42
Vitamin B_3	Whole blood	2/20	0/15

*Deficiency determined by comparison with each laboratory's reference standards. Since distribution of laboratories was nonrandom, comparison of mean values was not performed.

Two patients in the control group had serological evidence of chronic Epstein-Barr virus infection (NS), two were leukopenic, and none had transminase elevations.

Results of some nutritional parameters in both groups are presented in Table 1. The most prevalent findings were low blood levels of pyridoxal phosphate and magnesium. These were comparable in the two groups.

Analysis of essential fatty acids in serum and erythrocyte phospholipids was performed in 9 patients in each group. Low levels of 20:5 6 (eicosapentaenoate, EPA) were found in 6 patients with MCS and 5 controls. Elevations of 20:4 6 (arachidonate, AA) were found in 6 MCS and 3 controls (NS). Because different laboratories were used for the determinations and were unequally divided between the two groups, a comparison of mean values was not performed.

Fractionated, quantitative urine amino acid analysis was obtained in 29 MCS and 20 controls consuming standardized diets. The results are presented in Table 2. The most striking finding is the large proportion of MCS patients (41%) with very low excretion of essential amino acids compared to a 5% frequency of this occurrence in the control group ($x^2 = 8.54$, $p < 0.01$). Two of the MCS patients

Table 2. Amino Acid Excretion in MCS and Control Patients

FINDING	MCS N = 29	CONTROL N = 20
Normal excretion	7	13
Diminished excretion of 6 or more essential amino acids	12	1
Hyperaminoacidurias		
Ethanolaminuria	2	3
Taurinuria	3	2
Beta-aminoaciduria	2	1
Generalized, non-specific	3	0

with low excretion of essential acids were hypoalbumenic for no apparent reason. Serum albumen was 3.1 gm% in one and 1.9 gm% in another. Neither of these showed evidence of generalized malabsorption, proteinuria or liver disease. Both suffered from chronic nonspecific bowel complaints, as did all patients with low urinary excretion of essential amino acids, and many with normal excretion patterns.

Erythrocyte activity of superoxide dismutase (ESOD) was determined in 27 MCS and 19 controls. Diminished enzyme activity was found in 24 patients (89%) and 15 controls (79%) (NS).

Mean values of ESOD were 7.40 ± 2.44 units/mgHb in MCS group and 7.85 ± 3.43 units in the control group (NS). There was no association between ESOD activity and serum, urine, erythrocyte and hair copper levels in the few patients in whom those were measured.

Erythrocyte glutathione peroxidase activity (EGPx) was determined in 23 MCS and 14 controls. Results are presented in Table 3. The proportion of MCS patients with low EGPx (48%) is greater than the proportion of controls with low EGPx (36%); however, this difference is not significant and the mean values of EGPx are not significantly different between the two groups.

Lipid peroxides were measured in 8 patients, 6 with MCS and 2 controls. They were elevated in 4 MCS and 1 control. (ESOD, EGPx and lipid peroxide determinations were all performed by Monroe Medical Research Laboratory.)

DISCUSSION

The problem of MCS is associated with significant occupational morbidity. Sixty-four percent of the patients in this study had stopped work or made major career changes because of their illness; none of the control group had done so.

Considered as a group, patients with MCS tend to have a high prevalence of common physiologic disturbances. About one-fifth have thyroid disease, and an overlapping fifth have symptomatic mitral valve prolapse. The frequency of both these conditions was slightly higher in the MCS group than in the patient control group, but did not achieve statistical significance.

Undiagnosed hypothyroidism is found in over 10% of patients hospitalized for depression, and a history of thyroid disease is equally common in phobic patients.[18] Mitral valve prolapse occurs in 15–50% of patients with panic disorder.[13,19,32] Symptomatic prolapse is often associated with autonomic nervous system dysregulation, which may contribute to attacks of panic and poor exercise toler-

Table 3. Erythrocyte Glutathione Peroxidase (EGPx) Activity in MCS and Controls

	MEAN*	S.D.	LOW	NORMAL	HIGH
MCS	4.94	1.99	11	10	2
Controls	5.54	2.87	5	8	1

*μ Moles NAPH

ance.[3] The identification and treatment of occult thyroid disease or of autonomic dysregulation has been, in my experience, among the most rewarding clinical interventions in relieving symptoms associated with MCS. Patients do not necessarily report a decrease in hypersensitivity but experience a general increase in level of well-being.

Patients with MCS show numerous biochemical abnormalities. Most of these are common in patients with allergic illness and do not suggest a specific biochemical lesion as a cause of MCS. Low levels of pyridoxal phosphate (P-5-P) were equally prevalent in MCS and controls. Deficiency of P-5-P is common in asthma[26] where its appearance is independent of dietary Vitamin B_6. The administration of pyridoxine 200 mg/day was reported to improve asthma in such patients. Administration of high doses of vitamin B_6 may improve symptoms in MCS, especially when pyridoxal phosphate deficiency is present.

Magnesium deficiency was found in 31% of MCS and control patients. This is consistent with reports of Mg deficit in one-third of atopic patients.[6] Mg is an important modulator of immune function.[10] Its administration is protective in animal models of allergic sensitization.[10] Mg supplementation has recently been proposed to be beneficial in relieving the dysautonomic symptoms of patients with mitral valve prolapse.[11] For 10 of the MCS patients in this study (18%), oral or parenteral administration of Mg salts produced major improvement in a variety of symptoms, including fatigue, tachycardia, anxiety, insomnia, paresthesias and muscle spasm.

Abnormal metabolism of essential fatty acids (EFA) is a biochemical feature of atopic illness that may contribute to the appearance of immune dysfunction.[9] Low levels of eicosapentaenoate (EPA), found in both patient groups, is common. An unusual finding in patients with MCS is an elevation of circulating levels of arachidonic acid, the principle precursor of leucotrienes and prostaglandins. Nutritional supplementation with EPA from fish oils may benefit a number of symptoms associated with excessive prostanoid production or reactivity, including migraine headaches, arthritis, asthma, and dysmenorrhea.[9] It proved to be of marginal value in treatment of the MCS patients reported here, possibly because utilization of dietary EFAs requires normal nutritional status of copper[4] and selenium,[9] and these minerals appeared to be quite abnormal in these patients.

Erythrocyte superoxide dismutase is a copper-containing enzyme. Its activity is an index of copper status in experimental animals and humans.[22,28] SOD reduces damaging superoxide anions to H_2O_2, limiting inflammatory and toxic damage to the cells. Its full protective activity requires the cooperation of glutathione peroxidase (EGPx), which reduces H_2O_2 to H_2O.[5] Copper deficiency lowers SOD activity and may cause a compensatory increase in EGPx activity.

EGPx is a sensitive index of selenium status.[23,24] EGPx is depressed in patients with rheumatoid arthritis[30] and inflammatory skin diseases.[12] Selenium supplementation has been demonstrated to improve inflammatory symptoms in the former group.

ESOD and EGPx levels were generally low in MCS patients. Both defects appear to be reversible, as nutritional supplementation consistently raised levels of the enzymes toward normal. Copper deficiency is one of the few conditions that elevates tissue and blood arachidonate levels in animals and humans.[4] The distribution of low ESOD levels and of elevated arachidonate suggest that copper deficiency may be prevalent in both groups of patients, more so in MCS. Selenium deficiency (demonstrated by EPGx) is also highly prevalent in both groups and is slightly more likely to occur with MCS. Selenium deficiency increases the susceptibility of animals and humans to toxic effects of environmental pollutants[21,27] and fungal infections.[1]

The most striking difference between MCS and control patients lies in the unusually low excretion of essential amino acids in 40% of MCS patients who underwent urinary amino acid fractionation. Low excretion of amino acids despite a high protein diet may be due to several causes: (1) protein loss from body fluids; (2) increased utilization of amino acids for growth or repair; (3) maldigestion or malabsorption; (4) enhanced renal tubular reabsorption. No evidence of abnormal protein losses or high protein requirements for anabolic processes was present in these patients, although mild protein-losing enteropathy cannot be excluded. Hypoalbumenemia in 2 patients and clinical improvement with amino acid supplementation in 3 others suggests that amino acid needs were not being met by their high protein diets.

Sulfur-containing amino acids play a critical antioxidant role in inflammation.[8] Aromatic amino acids function as free-radical quenchers and as precursors of neurotransmitters. Further studies to define the pathophysiology of MCS should probably focus on disturbances in protein metabolism, since amino-acid excretion is the one area that clearly separates MCS from allergy.

SUMMARY AND CONCLUSIONS

Patients with MCS show numerous physiological and biochemical abnormalities and are generally sicker than a control group of allergic patients. Associated with MCS are mitral valve prolapse, hypothyroidism, autoimmune thyroiditis, specific abnormalities of amino acid and essential fatty acid metabolism, and diminished activity of ESOD and EGPx. Equally prevalent among MCS patients and controls are deficiencies of magnesium and Vitamin B_6.

Since patients with MCS feel sick almost all of the time, it is likely that some of these abnormalities contribute to their general level of ill health, if not to their sensitivities. It is also possible that these various abnormalities are caused by some unidentified fundamental metabolic or neuroendocrine disturbance that is common to states of hypersensitivity. A provocative finding is the high frequency with which impaired anti-oxidant levels were detected. Erythrocyte activity of SOD was low in 89% and EGPx was low in 48% of MCS patients. Furthermore, 41% showed impaired excretion of essential amino acids, despite a high protein diet, and leucocyte vitamin C was low in the 5 patients not taking vitamin C supplements. Anti-oxidant deficiences may certainly contribute to hypersensitivity to environmental pollutants and toxic chemicals. In fact, treatment with anti-oxidants, including selenium, vitamin C, copper, zinc, and sulfur-containing amino acids was associated with major clinical improvement in 14 (25%) of the patients in the MCS group and with limited relief of symptoms in another 10 (18%). In all patients in whom ESOD or EGPx were repeated, improvement in levels was observed following treatment. Therefore, it appears likely that the levels of these enzymes reflect dietary intake of selenium and copper, and that low enzyme levels could contribute to the pathophysiology of MCS. When compared with the data of Terr,[31] these findings indicate that a biochemical rather than immunologic basis for MCS is more likely. Protein metabolism in MCS deserves further investigation.

While allergic patients without MCS rarely showed the impairment in amino acid excretion seen with MCS, they often presented with low SOD or EGPx levels, and mean enzyme levels did not vary significantly between the two patient groups. Furthermore, half the MCS patients did not respond clinically to anti-oxidant supplementation, even if enzyme levels improved. It is therefore likely that other factors play significant roles in the genesis of the illness. Impaired excretion or catabolism of xenobiotics with their accumulation in body tissue[14] may complement defective anti-oxidant defenses in producing MCS.

REFERENCES

1. Boyne R, Arthur JR: The response of selenium-deficient mice to Candida albicans infection. J Nutr 116:816–822, 1986.
2. Brodsky CM: 'Allergic to everything': A medical subculture. Psychosomatics 24:731–742, 1983.
3. Coghlan C, Phares P, Cowley M, et al: Dysautonomia in mitral valve prolapse. Amer J Med 67:236–244, 1979.
4. Cunnane SC, Horrobin DF, Manku MS: Contrasting effects of low or high copper intake on rat tissue lipid essential fatty acid composition. Ann Nutr Metab 29:103–110, 1985.
5. Das SK, Nair RC: Superoxide dismutase, glutathione peroxidase, catalase and lipid peroxidation of normal and sickled erythrocytes. Br J Haematol 44:87–92, 1980.
6. Durlach J: Rapports expérimentaux et cliniques entre magésium et hypersensibilité. Rev Fr Allerg 5:133–146, 1975.
7. Feldman RG, Ricks NL, Baker EL: Neuropsychological effects of industrial toxins. Am J Indust Med 1:211–227, 1980.
8. Forman HJ, Rotman EI, Fisher AB: Role of selenium and sulfur-containing amino acids in protection against oxygen toxicity. Lab Invest 49:148–153, 1983.
9. Galland L: Increased requirements for essential fatty acids in atopic individuals: A review with clinical descriptions. J Amer Coll Nutr 5:213–228, 1986.
10. Galland L: Magnesium and immune function, an overview. Magnesium (in press).
11. Galland L, Baker SM, McLellan R: Magnesium deficiency in the pathogenesis of mitral valve prolapse. Magnesium 5:165–174, 1986.
12. Juhlin L, et al: Blood glutathione peroxidase levels in skin diseases: Effects of selenium and Vitamin E treatment. Act Dermatol-Venereol 62:211–214, 1982.
13. Kantor JS, Zitrin CM, Zeldis SM: Mitral valve prolapse syndrome in agoraphobic patients. Am J Psychiatr 137:467–469, 1980.
14. Laseter JL, DeLeon IR, Rea WJ, Butler JR: Chlorinated hydrocarbon pesticides in environmentally sensitive patients. Clin Ecol 11:3–12, 1983.
15. Levine SA: Oxidants/anti-oxidants and chemical hypersensitivities (Part one). Int J Biosocial Res 4(1):51–54, 1983.
16. Levine SA: Oxidants/anti-oxidants and chemical hypersensitivities (Part two). Int J Biosocial Res 4(2):102–105, 1983.
17. Levine SA, Reinhardt JH: Biochemical-pathology initiated by free radicals, oxidant chemicals,

and therapeutic drugs in the etiology of chemical hypersensitivity disease. J Orthomol Psychiatr 12:166–183, 1983.

18. Lindemann CG, Zitrin CM, Klein DF: Thyroid dysfunction in phobic patients. Psychosomatics 25:603–606, 1984.

19. Mavissakalian M, Salerni R, Thompson ME, Michelson L: Mitral valve prolapse and agoraphobia. Am J Psychiatr 104:1612–1614, 1983.

20. McCay PB, Gibson DD, Fong KL, Hornbrook KR: Effect of glutathione peroxidase activity on lipid peroxidation in biological membranes. Biochem Biophys Acta 431:459–469, 1976.

21. Mercurio SD, Combs GF: Selenium-dependent glutathione peroxidase inhibitors increase toxicity of prooxidant compounds in chicks. J Nutr 116:1720–1726, 1986.

22. Okahata S, Nishi Y, Hatano S, et al: Changes in erythrocyte superoxide dismutase in a patient with copper deficiency. Eur J Pediat 134:121–124, 1980.

23. Paglia DE, Valentine WN: Studies on the quantitative and qualitative characterization of erythrocyte glutathione peroxidase. J Lab Clin Med 70:158–169, 1967.

24. Perona G, et al: In vivo and in vitro variations of human erythrocyte glutathione peroxidase activity as result of cells aging, selenium availability and peroxide activation. Br J Haematol 39:399–408, 1978.

25. Rea WJ, Butler JR, Laseter JL, DeLeon IR: Pesticides and brain-function changes in a controlled environment. Clin Ecol 2(3):145–150, 1984.

26. Reynolds RD, Natta CL: Depressed plasma pyridoxal phosphate concentrations in adult asthmatics. Am J Clin Nutr 41:684–688, 1985.

27. Shakman RA: Nutritional influences on the toxicity of environmental pollutants. Arch Environ Health 28:105–113, 1974.

28. Solomons NW: Biochemical, metabolic and clinical role of copper in human nutrition. J Amer Coll Nutr 4:83–105, 1985.

29. Tappel AL: Selenium-glutathione peroxidase and vitamin E. Amer J Clin Nutr 27:960–965, 1979.

30. Tarp U, et al: Low selenium level in severe rheumatoid arthritis. Scand J Rheumatol 14:97–101, 1985.

31. Terr AI: Environmental illness: A clinical review of 50 cases. Arch Intern Med 146:145–149, 1986.

32. Venkatesh A, Pauls DL, Crowe R: Mitral valve prolapse in patients with anxiety neurosis. Clin Res 26:656, 1978.

33. Yagi K: Assay for serum lipid peroxide level and its clinical significance. Yagi K (ed): Lipid Peroxides in Biology and Medicine, 1983, pp 223–242.

JAMES E. CONE, MD, MPH
ROBERT HARRISON, MD, MPH
RANDY REITER, PhD, MPH

PATIENTS WITH MULTIPLE CHEMICAL SENSITIVITIES: CLINICAL DIAGNOSTIC SUBSETS AMONG AN OCCUPATIONAL HEALTH CLINIC POPULATION

Occupational health practitioners are encountering individuals in their practices who present with unusual diagnostic and therapeutic dilemmas. These patients are often labeled by themselves, or other clinicians, as "hypersensitive," "allergic," "hypersusceptible," or as manifesting an "environmental illness." Although many of these patients feel too sick to work, assessment of impairments, disability, and attribution or cause is hindered by the current lack of clear diagnostic criteria, frequent lack of industrial hygiene data, and inadequate tools to evaluate the extent of impairment. This situation often leads to frustration on the part of the occupational health clinician, resulting in summary judgments that the patient's problems are psychosomatic in origin, or simply of unknown type.

From the patient's point of view, he or she is often searching sincerely for assistance, which may be medical, psychosocial, or economic in nature. Often patients are subject to simultaneous stress and anxiety due to the perplexing nature of their symptoms, perceived inability to continue to work in an environment that apparently exacerbates their condition, and social pressures to continue to tolerate what may be severe but not externally evident symptoms such as headache, difficulty concentrating, nausea, severe fatigue, somatic pain, or dizziness. At the same time they face economic pressures from threats to their income and costs of medical care. The usually safe refuges such as home or office may be sources of potential aggravation of the symptoms, leading to dramatic changes in lifestyle, habitat, and social contact based on efforts to avoid exposures to potential irritants, intoxicants or allergens.

The patient may then may seek multiple medical evaluations and is likely to get multiple conflicting opinions. This is a result of the combination of lack of awareness of the problem on the part of some clinicians and varying beliefs regarding the organic as opposed to the psychological bases of the problem. As a result of frustration with a perceived lack of interest on the part of the traditional medical community in the problem, the patient may consult alternative medical

From the Occupational Health Clinic, San Francisco General Hospital, and the Occupational Medicine Clinic, University of California, San Francisco, San Francisco, California

Reprint requests to James E. Cone, MD, MPH, Occupational Health Clinic, San Francisco General Hospital, 1001 Potrero Avenue, San Francisco, CA 94110 practitioners, including homeopathists, clinical ecologists, or acupuncturists/herbalists.

Such workers may embark on an often expensive course of diagnostic testing, including complex immunologic testing and challenge testing, and therapeutic modalities, including intradermal injections, rotation diets, and strict avoidance of all known or suspected environmental symptom-provoking agents.

At some point, patients may seek the advice of an occupational medicine clinician or toxicologist, either through self-referral, medical referral from puzzled primary care providers, or for medicolegal evaluation to determine impairment and work-relatedness of their condition.

What is the clinical nature of this condition? How can an appropriate diagnosis be reached using tools readily available to the occupational health practitioner? What are the clinical implications of this disorder? These are the subjects of this paper, which will be explored through analysis of our experience in San Francisco and a critical review of some of the existing literature.

METHODS

In order to better characterize this syndrome, case records from the University of California, San Francisco, occupational health clinics were reviewed. Records of the 850 patients who consulted the SFGH Occupational Health Clinic (OHC) between January 1984 and October 1986 and the records of 400 patients who consulted the Occupational Medicine Clinic (OMC) at UCSF between 1984–1986 were reviewed to determine whether they met the following criteria for consideration as a case of multiple chemical sensitivities (MCS):

1. History of development of symptoms involving multiple organ systems subsequent to exposure at their workplace. Cases of well-defined allergic reactions to specific chemicals, like occupational asthma or hypersensitivity pneumonitis, were excluded.

2. History of recurrence of symptoms involving multiple organ systems following exposure to low levels of multiple environmental stimuli.

Case characteristics in the following areas were abstracted: demographic information, occupation, social history (alcohol and cigarette consumption), history of specific exposures if known, family history, history of development and types of symptoms during the initial episode or period, history of recurrence of symptoms and associated exposure types, past medical history (including allergies and medications), past evaluations, diagnoses, and treatment recommendations. Descriptive analytic methods were then used to characterize the cases that met the case definition.

The available medical literature relevant to this syndrome and the diagnostic testing used by clinical ecologists were reviewed. Finally, three diagnostic subsets were identified that may have prognostic or therapeutic implications.

RESULTS

CHARACTERISTICS OF CASES

A total of 13 patients, 9 women and 4 men, met the criteria for inclusion in this case series. The demographic characteristics of the cases are listed in Table 1. The age of onset ranged from 29 to 46 years of age, with most cases occurring among those 30–40 years of age. The mean age of the cases was 42.8 years. The women were slightly older (mean age of 44), on average, than the men (mean age of 40).

Occupations that were represented more than once included school teachers, custodians, and electronics assembly workers. However, other occupations as diverse as postmaster and hospital cafeteria worker were also represented. There were a total of five industrial workers, three school employees, two skilled trades workers, one hospital service worker, and two office workers.

REPRESENTATIVE CASE HISTORIES

Case I. Mr. A is a 30-year-old painter who had a history of low back pain and seasonal rhinitis. He worked for five years without problems, using multiple types of enamel-based, epoxy and latex paints, and using both spray and roller. Following a particularly heavy exposure to sprayed lacquers, he developed severe symptoms of headache, dizziness, palpitations, shortness of breath, severe sleepiness, numbness in the extremities, sweating, irritability and overwhelming fatigue. He was seen by his personal physician, who removed him from further exposure for a period of several weeks. During that time the initial symptoms mostly resolved. However, when he attempted to return to work, he noted recurrence of the symptoms after only minimal exposure for a brief period of time. Subsequently he noted

Table 1. Demographic Characteristics of Cases from an Occupational Health Clinic Population

#	SEX	AGE AT ONSET	AGE	OCCUPATION	INDUSTRY	DURATION OF EXP.
1.	F	29	34	Printer	Printing	10 yr.
2.	M	30	33	Painter	Home construction	5 yr.
3.	F	31	44	School teacher	Secondary school	1 mon.
4.	M	34	35	School custodian	Elementary school	4 yr.
5.	M	35	39	Chemical technician	Chemical mfg.	7 yr.
6.	F	36	39	School teacher	Elementary school	7 yr.
7.	F	37	39	PVC molding operator	Plastics Mfg.	1 yr.
8.	F	38	47	Electronics assembly	Electronics mfg.	7 yr.
9.	F	39	40	Office manager	Real estate	1 yr.
10.	F	42	45	Cafeteria worker	Hospital	4 yr.
11.	F	45	52	Postmaster	Postal service	2 yr.
12.	F	46	56	Electronics assembly	Electronics mfg.	4 yr.
13.	M	49	54	Electronics assembly	Electronics mfg.	2 mon.

symptoms of severe anxiety, headaches, weakness, difficulty with vision, concentration and fatigue after exposure to household cleansers, automobile exhaust, gas-powered furnaces, perfume and ambient-air pollution.

He was evaluated by an ear, nose, and throat physician who treated him with meclazine without improvement in his symptoms. He was referred to a "stress clinic" where he was treated with group therapy and Mellaril, which exacerbated his symptoms. He was then referred to our occupational health clinic for medicolegal evaluation. Physical examination was normal. Neuropsychological examination confirmed his history of anxiety and panic attacks, and found evidence of a mild but definite short-term memory loss. He has been treated with avoidance of provoking exposures and retrained in work not involving exposure to organic solvents. His attacks have gradually decreased in frequency and severity over 1½ years.

Case II.   Ms. B is a 34-year-old printer/offset press operator exposed for over 10 years to solvents used in cleaning printing presses and printers ink. She developed urticaria, severe headaches, disorientation, emotional lability, and short-term memory disorder subsequent to exposure to the press cleaning solvents. Initially these symptoms were present only after exposure at work and resolved away from work. However, after about 8 years of exposure she noted recurrence of symptoms of headache, nausea, short-term memory loss, disorientation, sore throat and shortness of breath, which were associated with exposure to household cleaning products, gasoline, new buildings, fresh newsprint, new carpets or felt-tipped marking pens.

She was seen by several physicians, without definitive diagnosis or treatment, and was referred to us for medicolegal evaluation after the severity of her symptoms had caused her to quit work. She had a past hisory of chronic sinusitis, nonspecific urethritis, and a motor vehicle accident. Her family history was remarkable only for childhood allergies in her siblings. Physical examination was normal. Complete neuropsychological evaluation confirmed disorientation, emotional lability and anxiety. Avoidance of further organic solvent exposure was recommended. She obtained work in another field and has had gradual diminution of her symptoms.

Case III.   Mr. C is a 50-year-old black electronics assembler. He was well except for a history of seasonal bronchial asthma until he began work in an electronics company, where he soldered printed circuit boards with a hand-held soldering gun and cleaned the boards with a fluorinated hydrocarbon solvent. After several weeks he developed bloating in the stomach, dry cough, shortness of breath, and decreased appetite.

Since that time he has had recurrent symptoms of loss of concentration, trembling and heart palpitations whenever he is exposed to air-conditioned buildings, colognes, nail polish, paints, fresh newsprint, operating copy machines, or the cleaning section of grocery stores.

Physical examination was normal with the exception of a slight resting tremor, and no wheezing was noted on forced expiratory maneuver.

Pulmonary function testing revealed a mild restrictive ventilatory defect which was felt to be due to obesity. He has been able to continue to work as a security guard and attempts to avoid any exposures to organic solvents or air-conditioned buildings, which provoke recurrent episodes of his symptoms lasting up to two weeks following each exposure.

Case IV. Mr. D. is a 34-year-old white male school custodian who was well with the exception of history of seasonal rhinitis until he noted the gradual onset of severe headache, nausea and dizziness associated with exposures to blackboard cleaners, and floor cleaning and waxing chemicals. He also noted memory difficulties, mood changes, and fatigue. These symptoms recurred when he was exposed to buildings heated with gas stoves.

He consulted a local physician who diagnosed environmental allergies and placed the patient on a yeast-free diet, acupuncture treatments, and homeopathic treatments. He was removed from further workplace exposure by his physician.

Physical examination revealed faint wheezing on forced expiration, a 1/VI systolic murmur at the left sternal border, and a normal neurological examination. Laboratory testing included a complete neuropsychological evaluation which revealed normal concentration, memory, cognitive and motor functions, but confirmed a significant depression.

Material safety data sheets on the many chemicals to which the patient was exposed were obtained and revealed multiple exposures to organic solvents, particularly ethylene glycol monobutyl ether, xylene and chlorinated hydrocarbons (not further defined).

He obtained retraining in another field without exposure to organic solvents, and the frequency of his attacks have diminished gradually over several years.

DESCRIPTIVE ANALYSIS

Exposures Associated with Onset of the Syndrome. The exposures which were reported at the time of the onset of the syndrome are listed in Table 2. Organic solvents were the most common type of exposure, associated with the development of symptoms in 11 of 13 cases. In addition, the other two cases had exposures to pesticides or carpet glue that may well have included solvents as carriers or ingredients. Most were exposed to complex mixtures of solvents combined with other chemicals. Duration of exposure associated with the onset of symptoms ranged from as short as a few minutes or days to as long as 10 years.

Symptoms Associated with Onset. The distribution of symptoms is listed in Tables 3A–C. The most common symptoms associated with the onset of the syndrome were headaches (10 cases), nausea (5 cases), sore throat and weakness (4 cases each).

Table 2.   Exposures Reported Associated With Onset of Multiple Chemical Syndrome

		TYPE OF EXPOSURE		
CASE #	SOLVENTS[1]	PESTICIDES[2]	AIR POLLUTION[3]	NEW MATERIALS[4]
1.	X			
2.	X			
3.	X	X		
4.	X			
5.	X			
6.	X		X	
7.	X		X	
8.	X			
9.	X			
10.	X	X		
11.		X		
12.				X
13.	X			

[1]Solvents including paint thinner, lacquer thinner, Danish oil xylene, printing ink/press cleaners, methylene chloride, developers, trichloroethylene, Freon, Velva-Sheen, mop treatment with petroleum distillates, paints, and glycol ethers.
[2]Pesticides including diaxinon, guthion, and other organophosphates.
[3]Air pollutants including hydrogen sulfide and copy machines.
[4]New materials including carpets.

Exposures Associated with Recurrence of Syndrome.   The exposures associated with recurrence of the syndrome are listed in Table 4. The types of exposures include organic hydrocarbon solvents, new materials, products of combustion, odorants and cleaners.

Past Medical History.   Four of the individuals had a history of thyroid disease either at the time of onset or in the past, and three of these four were taking thyroid replacement medications at the time of their initial visits to the clinic. Two had a history of hypertension treated with diuretics, and one had a history of asthma treated with long-acting theophylline and inhaler bronchodilators.

Seven of the individuals had been evaluated by clinical ecologists and four by allergists, with a wide range of diagnostic tests, medications and diets prescribed for them.

Laboratory Testing.   In view of the retrospective nature of this analysis, and referral after prior testing by other treating physicians, no standard laboratory evaluation was performed. Based on symptoms and signs of memory loss, personality change, difficulty with concentration, or other neuropsychological symptoms, we referred six of the cases for complete neuropsychological testing. Three of the cases had a pattern of mild to moderate short-term memory loss, associated with difficulty with calculation and spatial organization. Two had anxiety and panic disorders. One had depression alone without cognitive deficits.

Table 3A. Symptoms Reported Associated With Onset of Multiple Chemical Sensitivity Syndrome

Symptoms	1.	2.	3.	4.	5.	6.	7.	8.	9.	10.	11.	12.	13.
HEENT													
Headaches	X	X	X	X	X			X	X		X	X	X
Sore throat					X	X			X				X
Sinus					X		X						
Eye irritation			X						X				
Nasal stuffiness											X		
Eye focus difficulties											X		
Nasal soreness						X							
RESP													
SOB	X							X					
Cough			X		X								X
Wheeze			X		X					X			X
Chest tightness						X							

Table 3B. Symptoms Reported Associated With Onset of Multiple Chemical Sensitivity Syndrome

	1.	2.	3.	4.	5.	6.	CASE # 7.	8.	9.	10.	11.	12.	13.
GASTROINTESTINAL													
Nausea			X			X	X	X			X		X
Abdominal pain						X	X						X
Gas							X						
Vomiting											X		
Constipation							X						
Bloating						X							
Decreased appetite													
VESTIBULAR													
Dizziness	X												
Intoxication						X		X	X				X
NEURO/PSYCHOLOGICAL													
Memory			X					X					
Concentration	X												
Numbness	X		X								X		
Tremors	X										X		
Palpitation	X												
Body pain						X							
SKIN													
Urticaria		X											

Table 3C. Symptoms Reported Associated With Onset of Multiple Chemical Sensitivity Syndrome

	1.	2.	3.	4.	5.	6.	CASE # 7.	8.	9.	10.	11.	12.	13.
MOOD/PSYCH													
Fatigue	X									X	X		
Sleepiness	X										X		X
Depression								X					
Disorient	X												
Emot. labile		X										X	
Irritable	X												
Confusion			X										
METABOLIC/MUSCULO-SKELETAL													
Sweats	X												
Aches			X							X	X		
Weakness				X							X	X	
Arthralgias													
Muscle tightness													

Table 4. Exposures Reported Associated with Recurrence of Multiple Chemical Sensitivity Syndrome

CASE #	SOLVENTS	ODORANTS	AIR POLLUTION	NEW MATERIALS
1.		Perfume	Smog	
2.	Gasoline			Newspapers
3.				Stores
4.	Petrochemicals			Newspapers
5.	Hair spray		Cig. smoke	New clothes
6.		Perfume	Car exhaust	Leather
7.			Copiers	Printed books
8.			Gas stoves	
9.	Gasoline, felt pens, paint		Tar	
10.	Paint	Perfume		Office bldgs.
11.	Paint, cleaners	Scented soaps		Carpets
12.			Gas stoves	Glues
13.	Nail polish remover	Perfume		Stores

TYPE OF EXPOSURE

DISCUSSION

Von Pirquet coined the word "allergie" in 1905 to describe a state of altered response or reactivity to environmental factors not usually affecting most individuals.[61]

So-called "food factors" that caused respiratory, cutaneous and gastrointestinal symptoms were subsequently reported, largely in the pediatric age group. In 1931, Albert Rowe published a book that described in detail a multisystem disorder that was due to selected foods.[57] His patients were of all age groups and had a wide range of respiratory and nervous system symptoms. He developed the elimination diet as the primary therapeutic modality.

The term "familial nonreaginic food allergy" was coined by Arthur Coca in the 1940's.[8] Again, patients with a polysymptomatic disorder due to food were described, presumably due to nonimmunologic mechanisms. The pulse test, a measure of cardiovascular response to specific food challenges, was developed.[9]

By the 1950's the concept of challenge testing with suspect foods was further elaborated by Rinkel.[54] The rotary diversified diet was developed to allow consumption of certain food items without provoking symptoms.

Theron Randolph was largely responsible for broadening the concept of food allergy to include environmental exposures.[37] Specific adaptation was used by Randolph to describe a syndrome of addiction to food and environmental chemicals, with a cyclic pattern of withdrawal and craving followed by temporary relief of symptoms on re-exposure to the offending item,[38] resulting over time in a syndrome of chronically maladapted responses to food and chemical exposures. It is primarily these patients, in Randolph's view, that come to the attention of the physician.

In order to characterize a chronic syndrome in which a clear cause-and-effect relationship to specific exposures could be seen, Randolph developed the Environmental Control Unit or Ecologic Unit.[40,41,45] A carefully planned and constructed short-term residential setting, this facility is designed to allow withdrawal of the individual from all deleterious exposures within an almost totally pollutant- and synthetic-chemical-free environment.

After a several-day period, the patient is challenged with incitant foods, natural gas, rubber, plastic, synthetics, and other materials that were reported to result in exacerbation of symptoms. Symptom responses are recorded based on careful scrutiny by the observer and reporting by the patient.

Randolph has also described the role of indoor air pollution in relation to psychiatric symptoms.[42,43] Hydrocarbon and other petroleum derivatives are the major incriminants. A more recent publication reviewed the concept of cerebral hypersensitivity and reported cases of "allergies" due to indoor air exposures.[12]

The Society of Clinical Ecology was formed in the mid-1960's. Clinical ecology broadly defined is the study of an individual's reaction to his or her environment. "Allergy" is conceived of as an "altered reaction" without regard to specific immunologic mechanisms.[13] Randolph has summarized the history of clinical ecology in a recent review[44] and two books have reviewed this subject comprehensively.[3,13]

The concept of environmental illness has been used to describe the individual who has altered reactivity to the potentially toxic products of industrial society. Patient support organizations and self-help guides have been developed.[12,16]

There have been several recent critical reviews of clinical ecology and its evaluation methods. A recent task force of the California Medical Association concluded, based on review of the available literature and presentations by clinical ecology practitioners, that "no convincing evidence was found that patients treated by clinical ecologists have unique, recognizable syndromes, that the diagnostic tests employed are efficacious and reliable, or that the treatments used are effective."[7]

A recent case series by Terr[59] described 50 patients who had been previously evaluated and diagnosed by 16 different clinical ecologists as having environmental illness. Clinical histories and exposure to chemicals were reportedly so varied that no patterns of symptomatology were identified. In only 2 of the 50 were there reported improvement of symptoms following treatment.

IMMUNOTOXICOLOGY

The study of immune function related to environmental toxins or occupational exposure has been expanding in recent years.[29,62,35] Toxic effects of chemicals on immune responses generally have most relevance when they can be adequately demonstrated at exposure levels that prove to be nontoxic by other toxicologic techniques.[58]

Evaluation of alteration of the immune system by chemical substances is difficult and results are often contradictory. A variety of general factors in animal studies influence the immune response: humoral factors, immunosuppressive drugs, adjuvants, stress, host nutrition, age and infection. Methodological problems need to be addressed as well, such as dose timing and role of direct cytotoxicity. In view of the complexity of the immune system, multiple assay batteries must be conducted to properly evaluate the major components of the immune response.[58] Relevant immunologic parameters suitable for evaluating chemically-induced immunotoxicity have been developed by the National Institute of Environmental Health Sciences.[11]

Halogenated aromatics,[30] heavy metals,[58] and organochlorine pesticides[58] have been among the most well-studied immunotoxins in animals and show the most consistent effects. Examination of immune function for selected substances appears to provide additional data pertinent to defining toxicity at the cellular level and for subsequent standards-setting. The significance of individual tests results, however, is difficult to interpret, and is not sufficiently characterized clinically to use in individual diagnosis at the present time.

Human epidemiological data are relatively scant. For specific substances such as vinyl chloride, immune testing may be a useful adjunct to biological monitoring.[58,63] The patient with possible multiple chemical sensitivites may have exposures to potential immunotoxins. There are, however, currently few human data associating particular immunological abnormalities with specific low-level exposures of potential interest, and most of these are associated with exposure to 2,3,7,8-tetrachlorodibenzodioxin or tetrachlorodibenzofurans.

CLINICAL EVALUATION

The clinical diagnostic evaluation of the patient with potential multiple chemical sensitivities should be based on current concepts of toxicology and pathophysiology. Both immunotoxicological methods and other procedures to test for abnormal responses bear scrutiny in this regard.

TESTS FOR ALTERED SENSITIVITY

A number of tests have been used as measures of altered responsiveness in patients, mostly related to the diagnosis of food allergy.

Intracutaneous titration is the intradermal injection with aqueous extracts to detect the first dilution that initiates progressive wheal formation. This test has been proposed by Rinkel[55] as a means of determining initial and optimal dosage for allergen treatments. Controlled studies suggest that this may be useful in establishing allergen sensitivity in the evaluation of patients with ragweed pollen-induced hay-fever,[60] but its role in the evaluation of multiple chemical sensitivities is not clear.

Radioallergosorbent (RAST) titration for IgE antibody was developed by Wide[64] and is commercially available in modified form as a method for establishing immunotherapy dosage. It is more expensive than standard skin testing, and it is unclear at this time whether it offers substantially increased information.

Subcutaneous-intracutaneous provocative testing and neutralization were developed as an addition to the Rinkel titration method. They were initially used for the diagnosis of food allergy and later for the diagnosis of inhalant allergy. While there are no fully reported double-blind studies of these methods, there are two studies evaluating them. One used oral food challenge to evaluate positive intracutaneous provocation tests. Out of 193 positive intracutaneous provocations, 62% were confirmed on oral food challenge and 38% were not.[14] The reproducibility and validity of this method for diagnosis of food allergy has been challenged by Bronsky,[5] who reported on a study of hospitalized asthmatics who were skin-tested and observed to compare their symptoms during a control period. Unfortunately, this critical article is presented in abstract form without data, making evaluation difficult.

Sublingual provocative testing and desensitization methods were first used by homeopathic practitioners in the 19th century. Two studies have supported its use. The first, by King,[25] evaluated effects of sublingual provocation with food antigen compared with placebo on psychological symptoms. Symptom scores were reportedly statistically significantly higher after antigen exposures. The second study, by Mandell,[31] studied food antigens, inhalants and placebo effects on arthritis pain. A significant response to food and inhalants was noted. However, several multi-center double-blind studies have failed to confirm its usefulness in diagnosis of food allergy.[52,53] These studies have been criticized[36] for unexplained loss of subjects, lack of testing for known allergens, and high placebo response rate (50% in one study). One other negative report was presented only in a letter to the editor.[24]

The leukocytotoxicity test, the cytolysis of leukocytes, has been proposed as a method of diagnosis of allergy.[6] Physiologic mechanisms are not clear, and no consistent relation between results of this test and the presence of clinical food allergy has been demonstrated.

These methods have been critically reviewed by Grieco and the American Academy of Allergy.[1,17] Two additional tests have been used as well and deserve further comment.

Immunological Testing. McGovern and others have recommended measures of immune response in the study of patients with food and chemical sensitivity.[33,26,32,34] T-cell subpopulation counts, helper/suppressor ratios, immunoglobulins, and immune complexes are among the tests suggested.[34] The relevance of individual abnormalities in immune function to the clinical presentation and to other disease states is not known, nor do the authors of these reports present convincing data from control populations.

The International Union of Immunology Societies, in collaboration with the World Health Organization, defined the recommendations for immunological tests.[22] This was summarized by Ritts.[56] Immunological tests have been clinically useful for only a relatively small group of disorders where a specific abnormality is suspect. T- and B-lymphocyte subsets may be quite useful as tools of epidemiologic investigation but should not be viewed as diagnostic in an individual patient.[16]

The constellation of immune responsiveness testing is expensive, and, in our view, may be misleading. While it may have a role in evaluation of patients with food allergy, it currently has no well-defined role in the routine evaluation of the patient with possible multiple chemical sensitivities.

Environmental Challenge Testing.   As described above, the environmental unit was developed to challenge patients with environmental irritants in a pollutant- and synthetic-chemical-free setting. William Rea has published a number of articles reporting series of patients with clinical disorders related to environmental agents.[47,48,49,50,51] Various foods and chemicals such as pesticides, solvents, perfumes, dyes, synthetic fabrics and natural gas were suspect. Associated signs and symptoms were numerous. Each patient has his or her symptoms reproduced on exposure to the incriminated substance as well as to inhaled chemicals such as formaldehyde, chlorine and phenol. Individual cases were shown to have alterations in serum complement, eosinophils, T lymphocytes, and immunoglobulins on challenge testing.

Environmental challenge testing has not been well validated as specific or sensitive in any other well-designed controlled clinical trials. The dose of exposure and actual absorption of the test substances are uncertain, and the significance of fluctuations in immunological parameters in individual patients challenged with these materials is unclear.

Environmental challenge in this form, except as part of a research protocol, cannot be currently recommended in the evaluation of individual patients.

CONCLUSION

What then are useful methods for the diagnosis of the patient with MCS?

It is usually possible, by a combination of a detailed history, physical examination, and a few specific test procedures to define the nature of the problem for the concerned patient. A history of allergy, atopy or asthma should be sought. In the review of our 13 cases, only 3 had a clear atopic history, suggesting that an allergic predisposition was no more common in this series than in the general population.

A detailed occupational and environmental history is, of course, crucial for assessing potential chemical exposures. Industrial hygiene data, if available, may be useful in documenting the extent of exposure. Often, however, the recurrent syndrome is provoked by exposure levels that are low and certainly well within the current occupational exposure limits.

Physical examination should be performed with particular attention to the skin, head, ears, eyes, nose, throat, respiratory tract, gastrointestinal tract and nervous system (including careful mental status examination). Often, however, as in our series, the physical examination is completely normal.

Often the history and physical examination is sufficient to exclude as reasonable possibilities an allergic disorder or classic occupational disease. Further workup, suggested by the history of specific symptoms or findings on physical examination, may include bronchial challenge testing with histamine or metha-choline. Intradermal injection of standardized antigen extracts may be useful in confirming a suspected reaction to common environmental allergens, but positive allergy skin tests alone do not identify an occupational or environmental disease.

Neuropsychological testing by an experienced clinical neuropsychologist is most useful in the evaluation of patients with history of central nervous system symptoms or findings suggestive of cognitive or motor impairment on mental status examination.

DIAGNOSTIC SUBSETS

We have identified several diagnostic subsets among our population of MCS patients that have useful prognostic and therapeutic implications.

Psychoorganic Syndrome (POS). It has been recognized since the end of the 19th century that solvents can cause acute intoxication symptoms. A series of studies from Scandinavia have found impairments in neuropsychological functions among workers chronically exposed to lower levels of solvents. [19,20,21,23,27,28] A chronic toxic encephalopathy has been found in painters, including evidence of cerebral atrophy and abnormalities in performance on standard neuropsychological tests. [2]

Three in our case series of patients with multiple chemical sensitivities were found to have psycho-organic syndrome based on a history of chronic occupational solvent exposure, with symptoms of fatigue, deterioration of memory, personality changes of an aggressive or depressive type, and frequent headaches, combined with objective impairment on neuropsychological testing. These patients may respond favorably to psychological counselling or biofeedback forms of treatment.

Chemical Headaches. Chemical headaches have been defined by Raskin[46] as headaches associated with chemical exposures, typically with a migraine or "vascular" character, pulsatile in quality, which may be associated with symptoms of nausea, dizziness, diarrhea, tightness in the face and abdominal cramping. Chemicals that have been associated with chemical headaches include organic solvents, monosodium glutamate, nitrates, tyramine, and phenylethylamine.

Four in our case series had symptoms most consistent with the diagnosis of chemical headache. Differences between cases of chemical headaches and POS include shorter duration of exposure (1–4 years) for chemical headache cases (compared with 5–10 years for POS), and shorter duration of disability (0–1 years) as compared with 1–4 years for the POS cases. Chemical headache cases were also distinguished by a lack of neuropsychological impairment and fewer types of symptoms. All four cases were in nonsmokers, as compared with only 1 of three cases of POS. These patients usually responded to symptomatic treatment of the recurrent migraine-like headache episodes.

Acquired Solvent Intolerance. Recently a syndrome of acquired solvent intolerance has been described by Gyntelberg[18] in a case series of workers from Denmark. These workers had a history of exposure to organic solvents and subsequently developed extreme sensitivity to very low levels of solvents, with multiple symptoms including dizziness, nausea and weakness.

Six of the patients in our case series meet the criteria for acquired solvent intolerance. Duration of exposure for these patients ranged from as little as 2 months to over 7 years. Four out of the six worked in service occupations. Most have reduced or eliminated their responsiveness over time by avoidance of known initiating factors.

FUTURE STUDIES NEEDED

We have attempted in this case series to describe the range of exposures, symptoms, and associated conditions that are found among persons who meet the definition of multiple chemical sensitivities. Hopefully, future controlled prospective scientific investigations will yield more insight into the diagnosis, treatment, and long-term prognosis of patients with multiple chemical sensitivities. In the meantime, the occupational medicine physician is faced with patients with multiple symptoms associated with low-level exposure to common environmental stimuli. Simply denying that these patients have any organic basis for their symptoms, as some physicians have done in the past, does not serve the interests of these patients but merely adds to the high level of frustration that they already face. Alternatively, identifying those patients who may meet the criteria for one of the specific diagnostic subsets of multiple chemical sensitivities may aid in their treatment and help to identify those who have the best prognosis.

REFERENCES

1. American Academy of Allergy: Position statements—controversial techniques. J Allergy Clin Immunol 67:333, 1981.
2. Arlien-Soborg P, Bruhn P, Gyldensted C, et al: Chronic painters' syndrome: chronic toxic encephalopathy in house painters. Acta Neurol Scandinav 60:149–156, 1979.
3. Bell I: Clinical Ecology. Bolinas, CA, Common Knowledge Press, 1982.
4. Brodsky C: Allergic to everything: A medical subculture. Psychosomatics 24:731, 1983.
5. Bronsky E, Burkley D, Ellis E: Evaluation of the provocative food skin test technique. J Allerg Clin Immunol 47:104, 1971; [abstract].
6. Bryan WTK, Bryan MP: The application of in vitro cytotoxic reactions to clinical diagnosis of food allergy. Laryngoscope 70:810–815, 1967.
7. California Medical Association: Scientific Board Task Force on Clinical Ecology: A critical appraisal. West J Med 144:239–245, 1986.
8. Coca A: Familial Non-reaginic Food Allergy. Springfield, IL, Charles C Thomas, 1942.
9. Coca A: The Pulse Test. New York, Arco, 1956.
10. Dadd D, Levin A: A Consumer Guide for the Chemically Sensitive. San Francisco, 1982.
11. Dean JH, Luster M, Boorman C: Methods and approaches for assessing immunotoxicity: An overview. Env Hlth Persp 43:27, 1982.
12. Department of Consumer Affairs, State of California: Clean your room! Sacramento, CA, State of California, 1982.

13. Dickey LD: The food factor in disease: Its history and documentation. Clinical Ecology 2:65, 1982.
14. Draper L: Food testing in allergy: Intradermal provocative vs. deliberate feeding. Arch Otolaryng 95:160–171, 1972.
15. Environmental Illness Association, PO Box 5003, Berkeley, CA 94705.
16. Goodwin J: OKT3, OKT4 and all that. JAMA 246:947, 1981.
17. Grieco M: Controversial practices in allergy. JAMA 247:3106, 1982.
18. Gyntelberg F, et al: Acquired intolerance to organic solvents and results of vestibular testing. Am J Ind Med 9:363–370, 1986.
19. Hane MO, Axelson J, Blume C, et al: Psychological function changes among house painters. Scand J Work Env Hlth 3:91–99, 1977.
20. Hanninen H: Psychological picture of manifest and latent carbon disulphide poisoning. Br J Ind Med 28:374–381, 1971.
21. Hanninen H, Eskelinen L, Husman K, et al: Behavioral effects of long-term exposure to a mixture of organic solvents. Scand J Work Env Hlth 4:240–251, 1976.
22. IUES/WHO Working Group: Use and abuse of laboratory tests in clinical immunology: Critical considerations of eight widely used diagnostic procedures. Clin Exp Immunol 46:662, 1981.
23. Knave B, Anshelm-Olsson B, et al: Long-term exposure to jet fuel. II. A cross-sectional epidemiologic investigation on occupationally exposed industrial workers exposed to various solvents. Scand J Work Env Hlth 4:19–45, 1978.
24. Kailin E, Collier R: Relieving therapy for antigen exposure. JAMA 217:78, 1971 [letter].
25. King D: Can allergic exposure provoke psychological symptoms? A double-blind test. Bio Psychiat 16:3–17, 1981.
26. Levin A, et al: Immune complex mediated vascular inflammation in patients with food and chemical illness [abstract]. Ann Allergy 47:138, 1981.
27. Lindstrom K: Psychological performances of workers exposed to various solvents. Scand J Work Env Hlth 2:129–139, 1973.
28. Lindstrom K, Harkonen H, Hernberg S: Disturbances in psychological functions of workers occupationally exposed to styrene. Scand J Work Env Hlth 2:129–139, 1976.
29. Luster M, Dean J, Moore J: Evaluation of immune functions in toxicology. *In* Hayes AW [ed]: Principles and methods of toxicology. New York, Raven Press, 1982.
30. Luster M, Faith R, Clark G: Laboratory studies on the immune effects of halogenated aromatics. Ann NY Acad Sci 320:473, 1979.
31. Mandell M, Conte A: The role of allergy in arthritis, rheumatism and polysymptomatic cerebral, visceral and somatic disorders: A double-blind study. J Int Acad Prev Med July 1982, pp 5–6.
32. McGovern JJ: Correlation of clinical food allergy symptoms with serial pharmacological and immunological changes in the patients plasma [abstract]. Ann Allergy 44:57, 1980.
33. McGovern JJ: The role of naturally-occurring haptens in allergy [abstract]. Ann Allergy 47:123, 1981.
34. McGovern JJ, et al: Clinical evaluation of the major plasma and cellular measures of immunity. J Orthomolecular Psych 12:60, 1983.
35. Moore J: The immunotoxicology phenomenon. Drug and Chemical Toxicology 5:67, 1979.
36. Podell RN: Intracutaneous and sublingual provocation and neutralization. Clin Ecol 11:13–20, 1983.
37. Randolph TG: Human ecology and susceptibility to chemical environment. Springfield, IL: Charles C Thomas, 1962.
38. Randolph TG: The specific adaptation syndrome. J Lab Clin Med 48:934, 1956.
39. Randolph TG: Specific adaptation. Ann Allergy 40:333, 1978.
40. Randolph TG: The ecologic unit. Hospital Management, 1964.
41. Randolph TG: Ecologic orientation in medicine: Comprehensive environmental control in diagnosis and therapy. Ann Allergy 23:7, 1965.
42. Randolph TG: Depressions caused by home exposures to gas and combustion products of gas, oil and coal. J Lab Clin Med X:942, 1955.
43. Randolph TG: Domicillary chemical air pollution in the etiology of ecologic mental illness. Int J Social Psych 16:243, 1970.
44. Randolph TG: Emergence of the specialty of clinical ecology. Clinical Ecology 2:65, 1982.
45. Randolph TG: Dynamics diagnosis and treatment of food allergy. Otol Clin North Am 617:7, 1974.
46. Raskin NH: Chemical headaches. Ann Rev Med 32:63–71, 1981.
47. Rea WJ: Environmentally triggered thrombophlebitis. Ann Allergy 37:101, 1976.

48. Rea WJ: Environmentally triggered small vessel vasculitis. Ann Allergy 38:245, 1977.
49. Rea WJ: Environmentally triggered cardiac disease. Ann Allergy 40:243, 1978.
50. Rea WJ: Food and chemical susceptibility after environmental overexposure: Case histories. Ann Allergy 41:101, 1978.
51. Rea WJ: Recurrent environmentally triggered thrombophlebitis: A five year followup. Ann Allergy 47:338, 1981.
52. Report of the Food Allergy Committee on the sublingual method of provocative testing for allergy, April 12, 1973. Ann Allergy 31:382–385, 1973.
53. Report of the Food Allergy Committee of the American College of Allergists on the clinical evaluation of the sublingual provocative testing method for diagnosis of food allergy. Ann Allergy 38:185–191, 1974.
54. Rinkel HJ, Randolph TG, Zeller M: Food Allergy. Springfield, IL, Charles C Thomas, 1951.
55. Rinkel HJ: Inhalant allergy: I. The whealing response of the skin to serial dilution testing. Ann Allergy 7:625–630, 1949.
56. Ritts R: Clinical utility of immunologic tests. Ann Int Med 96:779, 1982.
57. Rowe A: Food allergy: Its manifestations, diagnosis and treatment. Philadelphia, Lea, 1931.
58. Sharma [ed]: CRC Immunotoxicology, Volumes 1, 2. 1981.
59. Terr AI: Environmental illness: A clinical review of fifty cases. Arch Int Med 146:145–149, 1986.
60. Van Metre TE Jr, Adkinson NF Jr, Lichtenstein LM, et al: A controlled study of the effectiveness of the Rinkel method of immunotherapy for ragweed pollen hay fever. J Allergy Clin Immunol 65:288–297, 1980.
61. Von Pirquet C: Allergie. Munch Med Wochenschr 52:1457, 1906.
62. Vos JG: Immune suppression as related to toxicology. CRC Toxicology 5:67, 1977.
63. Ward AM, et al: Immunological mechanisms in the pathogenesis of vinyl chloride disease. Br Med J 1:936, 1976.
64. Wide L, Bennich H, Johansson SGO: Diagnosis of allergy by an in vitro test for allergen antibodies. Lancet 2:1105–1108, 1967.

RICHARD S. SCHOTTENFELD, MD

WORKERS WITH MULTIPLE CHEMICAL SENSITIVITIES: A PSYCHIATRIC APPROACH TO DIAGNOSIS AND TREATMENT

During a tour of a specialty metal parts manufacturing concern, I interviewed an employee whose job was to wire electronic circuitry. Other employees had suggested that I speak to her because of her remarkable ability to detect solvent leaks, breakdowns in the exhaust system, or the escape of any noxious or toxic fumes. She detected these fumes long before anyone else noted them and was reputed to be almost invariably accurate in detecting fumes—she sounded few or no false alarms. When I spoke to her, she seemed somewhat embarrassed by what she regarded as her increased susceptibility to being overcome by solvents or noxious odors. She assumed that her coworkers barely tolerated her idiosyncracies and probably made fun of her for what she regarded as her weakness. She suspected that they regarded her as being crazy, and she even had some suspicion that they were right in that judgment of her. After all, she felt light-headed and queasy, and she experienced headache, nasal congestion, and throat irritation following the least exposure to a variety of unpleasant odors.

The worker was thankful that she was able to leave her usual work station whenever she began to feel symptomatic. At these times, she was allowed to work in the business office, which was set off from the manufacturing area, until the odor had dissipated. She was also thankful that her coworkers tried to discover and eliminate the source of the odor. Although she also experienced symptoms outside of work in reaction to a variety of common environmental odors, she regarded her symptoms as relatively insignificant and had never consulted a doctor about them. She was somewhat surprised and perhaps even relieved when I suggested that perhaps her coworkers valued her ability to detect leaks before they received larger exposures and possibly became sick themselves.

The woman suffers from multiple chemical sensitivities (MCS). She has experienced an array of somatic symptoms after exposure to many different types of chemicals and odors at levels that a traditional toxicologist would view as *far* below the levels known or postulated to cause any discernible effect. A recognized allergy to a single compound or closely related group can not be invoked to explain her symptoms, because exposure to so many different types of substances brings about symptoms. Although in many respects she is quite similar to the other workers with MCS discussed in this volume, she differs from them in at least two important respects. Unlike these other workers, she

From the Department of Psychiatry, Yale University School of Medicine, New Haven, Connecticut

Reprint requests to Richard S. Schottenfeld, M.D., Yale University School of Medicine, 34 Park Street, New Haven, CT 06519.

has never consulted a physician for her symptoms, and she does not suffer any significant disability as a result of her symptoms. Since community surveys consistently identify that the majority of individuals with both somatic and psychological symptoms do not seek treatment for their symptoms, in order to understand the not inconsiderable disability associated with MCS we need to consider the question "what makes one person 'well' while other individuals with similar chemical sensitivities are 'ill?' "[9]

The relationship between chemical exposure, on the one hand, and pathophysiologic changes, symptoms, and illness in individuals with MCS, on the other hand, is a subject of much controversy, as is evident from this volume, but the more general relationship of pathophysiologic changes, symptoms, and illness is also problematic. Even in relatively well-understood medical diseases, there may be no one-to-one correspondence (isomorphism) between symptoms and pathophysiologic processes.[24] Some patients with severe impairment of pulmonary function, for example, may remain asymptomatic, while others with less severe impairment may be severely disabled by their symptoms, and studies of patients with peptic ulcer disease document that some patients with healed ulcers remain symptomatic while other patients with persistent ulcers become free of symptoms.[16]

Because the disparity between the severity of symptoms and the paucity of pathophysiologic findings in individuals with MCS is so great, some authors have suggested that the disorder can best be classified as one of a group of disorders known as "somatoform" (i.e., disorders in which physical symptoms suggest physical disorders but for which there are no demonstrable organic findings or known physiological mechanisms)[4]—idiopathic chronic pain syndromes are the most commonly occurring somatoform disorders in the United States.[11] The most recent classification of psychiatric disorders limits the use of the term "somatoform disorder" to conditions in which psychological factors are known or presumed to be of etiologic importance.[1] In the following section I will discuss the evidence suggesting that psychological factors are significant in leading to or perpetuating symptoms and disability in individuals with MCS.

In my view, individuals with MCS, like individuals with other somatoform disorders, comprise a heterogenous grouping. Some may have unusual sensitivities to a broad array of chemicals, although probably not on a strictly allergic or immunologic basis; some may amplify normal bodily sensations, which they incorrectly attribute to chemical exposure; some may amplify normal or mild irritant reactions to many environmental substances and become ill rather than only mildly symptomatic; other may suffer from primary psychiatric disorders; finally, some may suffer from psychiatric disorders secondary to MCS that further exacerbate symptoms and disability. In most cases, biological, psychological, social and cultural factors will all play important roles in affecting the illness of individuals with MCS. The second section of this paper will discuss the role that biological vulnerability or unusual sensitivity to chemicals plays in the disorder and will examine the roles that psychological, social and cultural factors play in affecting the perception, persistence, and amplification of symptoms. The third section will discuss the psychiatric disorders most often associated with patients with MCS, and the final section will discuss the implications of these psychological processes and psychiatric diagnoses for treatment of individuals with MCS.

Symptoms and Their Relation to Exposure

UNUSUAL SENSITIVITIES

Some individuals may have extremely low thresholds either for perceiving odors or for other indices of exposure, or for experiencing irritation of mucosal, dermal or neural tissue. That there is considerable variation from one person to the next in the acuity or sensitivity of the various perceptual systems (auditory, visual, tactile, olfactory and taste) should come as no surprise—one need only consider the different thickness and prisms of eyeglasses assembled at scientific meetings or other social functions. Laboratory studies document the extent of variation in odor detection as well as the extent to which different individuals experience symptoms of mucosal irritation when exposed to various noxious or toxic substances, such as cigarette smoke. Historical, social and environmental factors, in addition to genetic factors, may contribute to these differences, so that the same individual may be more or less sensitive at different times, depending on these factors. Rather than diminish, symptoms tend to increase the longer an individual remains exposed to noxious odors, e.g., non-smokers tend to have lower odor thresholds as well as lower thresholds for mucosal irritation than smokers.[6] Biological vulnerability to symptom development may be increased in certain pathophysiologic conditions. Asthmatic patients have long recognized that asthmatic symptoms may be exacerbated by exposure to the odor of perfumes or cologne, insecticides, household cleaning agents, cigarette smoke, fresh paint, automobile exhaust or gas fumes, and cooking smells. A recent study has documented decreases in FEV 1 of asthmatic patients exposed to minute concentrations of perfumes.[23] In addition, perceptual and symptomatic thresholds tend to be lowered in states of increased arousal or attentiveness, such as accompany exposure to novel situations, and thresholds are also lowered by anxiety and by expectations about exposure or symptoms.[24]

What is the relevance of these studies for understanding MCS? Clinically, I have been impressed by the facility and frequency with which individuals with MCS will both become symptomatic and accurately identify the lingering odor of furniture polish or paint in my office—odors that I can detect after these individuals bring them to my attention (aided by my memory of the strong odor accompanying the initial use of these substances) but which, at least most of the time, don't cause me any difficulties. It is not clear whether odor detection precedes symptoms, occurs simultaneously with or follows perception of symptoms. The study of asthmatics, discussed above, documents decreases in forced expiratory volumes following exposure to cologne even when odor detection is blocked by nasal occlusion, suggesting that at least some symptoms may occur independent of odor detection and the higher cortical reactions to odor detection. Whatever the physiologic sequence, however, it seems likely that individuals with MCS fall within the portion of the population with the lowest threshold for perception of odors and for experiencing irritative symptoms from chemicals.

AMPLIFICATION OF SYMPTOMS

The typical symptoms experienced by individuals with MCS (nasal congestion, throat or eye irritation, hoarseness, nausea, chest pain, palpitations, dyspnea, choking or smothering sensations, tremulousness, headache, light-headedness, dizziness, faintness, fatigue, and feelings of unreality) are relatively ubiquitous in the general population. A National Center for Health Statistics (NCHS) national survey, for example, found that 78% of Americans reported being bothered by at least one of 12 common symptoms, such as headache, palpitations, or dizziness,[14] and studies of college students are consistent with this finding.[15] Many of the symptoms of MCS are also the known physiologic concomitants of anxiety and fear. Symptoms related to hyperactivity of the autonomic nervous system, including tachycardia and palpitations, dyspnea, flushing, dry mouth, dizziness, light headedness, paresthesias, upset stomach, and diarrhea are normally experienced by individuals exposed to frightening or anxiety-provoking situations, and fatigue may follow these situations.

Individuals with MCS may differ from other individuals in their response to commonly occurring symptoms. Most people experience these symptoms only transiently and then dampen their response—they dismiss the symptoms as insignificant and divert their attention to other matters. Individuals with MCS, however, become increasingly anxious and aroused and symptomatic following the onset of symptoms—i.e., they tend to amplify rather than dampen their symptoms.

Amplification of symptoms may play a part in the genesis of the disorder of MCS regardless of whether the individual is unusually sensitive to chemicals or has even been exposed to toxic or noxious chemicals. The initial symptomatic episode for some individuals with MCS may be a direct result of chemical exposure; for others, the initial symptoms may be the symptoms of autonomic hyperactivity resulting from the fear associated with potential exposure; and for others, symptoms unrelated to any chemical exposure may be mistakenly attributed to exposure. Regardless of the initial etiology, the failure to dampen irritative symptoms or to modulate symptoms of anxiety may lead to profound disability associated with MCS.

Situational factors as well as personality or cognitive styles can predispose an individual to amplify bodily sensations and somatic symptoms.[3] Individuals are more likely to pay attention to their internal state (and consequently to amplify bodily sensations) when the external environment is monotonous or boring or when the environment is considered to be dangerous (e.g., following exposure to an unknown chemical). It is notable that these situations are quite typically found to be associated with the onset of symptoms of chemical sensitivities.

Expectancies and interpretive sets also affect the likelihood that symptoms will be amplified rather than dampened. Once symptoms are believed to be indicative of disease (rather than reflecting normal alterations in somatic functioning) or believed to be related to exposure to toxic chemicals, individuals are likely to become increasingly anxious (and symptomatic) following the initial detection of what might otherwise be considered (and dismissed) as relatively mild symptoms. Since expectancies, cognitive processing of symptoms, and interpretive sets play an important part in determining the individual's response to symptoms and disease regardless of the etiology of symptoms (i.e., even if physiologic changes and symptoms are caused directly by exposure to chemicals), the individual's cognitive processing and interpretive set will affect his or her response to these symptoms and illness behavior. I will discuss these factors in greater depth in what follows.

Detection of an odor, perception of other indices of exposure, or perception of somatic changes or symptoms are only the first steps in a sequence of cognitive processing that culminates in illness. Solvent intoxications provide a useful example. Although symptoms of intoxication (including light-headedness and alterations in consciousness) are experienced almost universally at sufficiently high exposures to a variety of organic solvents,[21] some individuals enjoy the experience and seek out reexposure while others feel terrified by the experience and dysphoric. Some of the differences between those who enjoy the high and those who become sick from exposure may reflect differences in biological susceptibility or the differential sensitivity of various organ systems or neural systems to exposure (e.g., exposure may directly cause overactivation of neural systems regulating anxiety in individuals who become sick, whereas these systems may be activated only to the point of heightened arousal and pleasurable excitation in individuals who enjoy the high). Expectations about the effects of exposure and interpretations about the significance of these effects may also affect how anxious and dysphoric the person becomes—those who expect to enjoy the high and deliberately reexpose themselves are more likely to feel euphoric than are those who regard any alteration in consciousness as a sign of illness and who are exposed unwillingly.

The etiology and significance of symptoms are often unclear, and interpretation of symptoms will depend on a person's previous experience with similar sensations, the context in which symptoms occur, interpersonal communications, and information available about the situation.[3,19,20] Once formed, interpretive sets tend to persist—humans tend to search for confirmatory evidence and to disregard discrepant information. Interpretive sets also influence the perception of subsequent sensations. Depending on the interpretive set, an individual may be more or less distressed by the same physiologic event, and neutral events may be perceived as either pleasurable or painful depending on the individual's expectations. Rodin's example is illustrative of the significance of an interpretive set.[19] Once someone has been told that she or he looks ill, then normal shortness of breath following exertion may be taken as further evidence of sickness, and actions taken to avoid symptoms, such as walking more slowly, may further strengthen the individual's sense that she or he is ill. Anxiety about being ill might further exacerbate symptoms (shortness of breath, palpitations, chest pains), leading to a cascade of increasing conviction about illness, increasing anxiety, increasing symptoms, and increasing disability.

A similar sequence probably accounts for illness in at least some patients considered to have MCS. Regardless of the original etiology of symptoms of chemical sensitivities, anxiety will augment these symptoms, and, once someone begins to interpret symptoms as being indicative of toxic exposure, both anxiety and symptoms will increase. The relatively more frequent development of chemical sensitivities in situations of realistic potential exposure to toxic substances (e.g., the workplace), where individuals are more anxious and more vigilant to discover evidence of "toxicity" in themselves than they are in non-threatening environments, is consistent with this hypothesis. Increased awareness of the possible harmful effects of exposure, such as occurs following dissemination of information about toxic hazards, would also be expected to increase the incidence of the disorder, and this also seems to be a frequent finding in the history of individuals with MCS. It would be a mistake, however, to conclude from this that information about potential health hazards should be suppressed. Transient hypochondriasis in medical students results from a similar process,[12,24] and, for both hypochondriasis in medical students and symptoms of MCS, provision of additional information by a reliable, trusted, and well-informed expert, in a reassuring manner, may be more likely than suppression of information to ameliorate symptoms and anxiety.

The tendency of interpretive sets, once formed, to persist explains some of the tenacity with which individuals hold on to their perhaps mistaken beliefs and misattributions about symptoms and illness. Reassurance alone, without substitution of an alternative and believable interpretive set, is likely to be futile. Even provision of a substitute interpretive set may be ineffective when the individual's interpretive set is well-established, consistent with earlier experiences of illness, and supported by family, friends, or medical experts. Additionally, when the rewards of continued belief in the original interpretive set and continued illness (i.e., the sick role and the secondary gains of illness, such as increased caring from others and relief from family, social, and work obligations) outweigh the benefits of healthy functioning, both the interpretive set and illness are also likely to persist.

GENERALIZATION OF SYMPTOMS

One of the characteristic features of the disorder of MCS is that symptoms, which initially occur only in response to circumscribed exposures to discrete substances, eventually are provoked by exposure to many different types of chemicals and odors. One way of understanding this feature of MCS is to view symptoms of MCS as a learned response to noxious exposures and to view the ever-widening array of exposures that cause symptoms as a result of primary stimulus generalization. Campbell, et al. (1964) demonstrated that marked anxiety reactions (the conditioned response) can be conditioned by a single severe stress (the unconditioned stimulus, in this example, respiratory paralysis induced by succinylcholine). Repeated evocation of the conditioned response by the conditioned stimulus (a pure, neutral tone), even in the absence of the unconditioned stimulus, was accompanied by increased strength of response rather than by extinction.[7] One might hypothesize that MCS could similarly be induced by an initial traumatic exposure. Primary stimulus generalization would result in a wide range of tones producing the conditioned response. An alternative way of understanding the generalization of symptoms in MCS is to use a somewhat more intuitively satisfying, combined cognitive and behavioral model. Generalization of symptoms results from the individual's mistaken cognitive appraisal that odors that resemble the initial traumatic exposure will be equally dangerous. In this view, individuals with MCS essentially scare themselves into having symptoms of anxiety as a result of expecting this occurrence after detecting an odor, and the repeated occurrence of symptoms following exposure reinforces the learned response.

DEVELOPMENTAL FACTORS RELATED TO MULTIPLE CHEMICAL SENSITIVITIES

As with idiopathic chronic pain syndromes and other somatoform disorders,[2] the early childhood history of individuals with MCS is often notable for the presence of physical or sexual abuse, severe medical illness during childhood, death of one or both parents, or other severe disturbances of early care-giving relationships. Considering the importance of cognitive processing of symptoms and of the ability (or lack thereof) to soothe oneself in the genesis and maintenance of the disorder, the history of severe disruptions in early care-giving relationships of individuals who go on to develop MCS is perhaps not surprising. The ability to soothe oneself, to modulate anxiety, or to dampen the physiologic responses to anxiety-provoking stimuli is at least partially learned (or not learned) in the interactions with caregivers. The cognitive ability to interpret correctly the meaning and significance of somatic symptoms or bodily states must also be learned in early childhood through interactions with caregivers (consider, for example, the process of learning to identify hunger as a distinct state from other states of distress—the process begins with the caregiver learning to distinguish between the child's cry motivated by hunger and the cries motivated by other discomfort—for a full discussion, cf. ref. 5[5]). The increasingly anxious and frantic response of individuals with MCS when "trapped" in a hostile or "toxic" environment may represent a repetition of early failures to ameliorate distress in a consistent manner. The cascade of symptoms provoked by minor exposures in individuals with MCS thus reflects both a long-standing personality deficit (i.e., a failure to learn to interpret correctly distress and to soothe onself) as well as a more recently learned, pathologic response to noxious stimuli.

PSYCHIATRIC DISORDERS AND MULTIPLE CHEMICAL SENSITIVITIES

Until now, this paper has emphasized the considerable role that the cognitive processing of symptoms and that a particular affective state, anxiety, play in affecting symptoms and disability associated with MCS. This section will discuss the relationship between MCS and specific psychiatric disorders, including affective disorders (depression and anxiety disorders) and other somatoform disorders (hypochondriasis, somatization disorder or hysteria, and conversion disorders).

The recent report by Terr (1986) that 31 of 50 patients (62%) previously diagnosed by clinical ecologists to be suffering from environmentally induced illness had, for many years, experienced many symptoms involving multiple systems and parts of the body "most likely of psychological origin" suggests a need to define the psychiatric disorders experienced by individuals with MCS.[25] Since epidemiologically sound diagnostic studies of individuals with MCS have not yet been undertaken, the discussion that follows will of necessity be somewhat anecdotal and speculative.

CHEMICAL SENSITIVITIES, DEPRESSION AND ANXIETY

Although depression is one of the most pervasive disorders confronting medical practitioners in any clinical setting, it is also one of the least well diagnosed and treated conditions. Community surveys document six-month prevalence for affective disorders ranging between 6.1 and 9.5% in the general population.[18] Depressed individuals often experience a variety of somatic symptoms in association with their depression, seek medical care more often than individuals without any psychiatric disorders, and are more likely to seek medical care in general medical clinic settings than in mental health facilities.[17] Surveys of medical clinic populations identify between 10 and 40% of ambulatory medical patients as depressed, and these surveys also document that depression is not routinely diagnosed or treated in these patients.[13]

One explanation for the increased utilization of medical care services and underutilization of psychiatric services by depressed individuals and for the failure to diagnose and treat depression in these individuals is that the usual hallmarks of depression (pervasive sadness, depressed mood, and tearfulness) are often absent or inconspicuous for many depressed individuals. Instead, these depressed individuals predominantly experience cryptogenic somatic complaints or neurotic symptoms such as anxiety, phobias, and obsessions. Historically, the term "atypical depression" has been used for the diagnosis of such individuals.[8] Rather than feel sad or depressed, individuals with atypical depression complain of relatively nonspecific somatic symptoms, many of which overlap with the symptoms experienced by individuals diagnosed as suffering from MCS. Individuals with atypical depressions are aware that something is wrong with them, but they experience or focus primarily on the somatic signs and symptoms of disease and not on their emotional state. Regardless of whether these individuals have a distinctive neurochemical or biological basis for experiencing an atypical form of depression or whether they somatize (i.e., tend to perceive or focus exclusively on medical or somatic symptoms rather than recognize emotional, psychological, or psychiatric difficulties) on the basis of individual psychological or historical factors or because of social and cultural influences, atypical depression and major depression appear to be closely related or overlapping disorders. Vegetative signs and symptoms of depression, such as disorders of sleep, appetite, and libido, disturbances in social functioning, and loss of interest in usual activities are common in both atypical and typical major depression. In addition, individuals with atypical depression often have a family history of depression, often go on to develop a typical major depression, and tend to respond favorably to antidepressant medications.

A brief clinical vignette will illustrate the role that major depression may play in MCS:

Mrs. A., a 46-year-old, married, white woman, who was exposed at work to spray paints, including epoxy resins and accelerators, experienced recurrent episodes of coughing, chest tightness, throat and eye irritation, and nasal and sinus congestion for about one year before experiencing a particularly severe episode during which she felt extremely anxious and apprehensive. Asthma, rhinitis, and sinusitis were diagnosed on the basis of physical and radiological examination and pulmonary function tests. Despite removal from work and vigorous medical treatment, she experienced persistent symptoms, often triggered or exacerbated by exposure to perfumes, household cleaners, or atmospheric pollution. She became increasingly preoccupied about her medical symptoms and feared that she would never recover her health. Eventually she was referred for psychiatric evaluation. Although she focused on her medical symptoms, she acknowledged that she had become increasingly sad, irritable and anxious. She had also developed a fear of driving her car, had lost interest in most of her usual activities, and was experiencing chronic sleep difficulties and difficulties with memory and concentration. She appeared to be depressed.

Mrs. A. was reluctant to begin a trial of antidepressant medication, but she agreed to a participate in a time-limited (ten-session) psychotherapy. During the course of psychotherapy, Mrs. A. discussed her fears about the possibility of reexposure at work and her disappointment and resentment that her supervisor had not done anything to protect her from exposure even after she began to complain of difficulties. She developed plans to express her anger through a grievance procedure and through increased involvement in her union. She also came to recognize that a number of longstanding family problems contributed to her anxiety and depression and that when she was working she was better able to cope with these problems. Finally, she was relieved that a new exhaust system was installed at work. As she became aware of how much her symptoms were amplified by her fears, anxiety, anger and depression, she began to anticipate the difficulties she might encounter when she returned to work and to densensitize herself to her anticipated fears. While still in therapy, she returned to work. Her initial exacerbation of symptoms after returning to work was managed jointly by the psychiatrist and internist. Although she continues to experience recurrent episodes of rhinitis and sinusitis, her symptoms are managed relatively well with standard medical treatments, and she has suffered little additional disability.

The crucial role of anxiety in leading to and perpetuating symptoms of MCS has been discussed above. Several well-defined and relatively discrete anxiety disorders, including generalized anxiety disorder, panic disorder, and post-traumatic stress disorders, deserve special mention because of the possibility that these disorders are sometimes mistaken for MCS.

Individuals with panic disorders experience frequent episodes (at least three times within three weeks) of panic attacks that are unrelated to marked physical exertion or to exposure to a life-threatening situation or a circumscribed phobic stimulus. Panic attacks are manifested by discrete periods of apprehension and fearfulness and are accompanied by at least four of the cognitive or autonomic symptoms of anxiety listed above and noted to overlap with symptoms that are often attributed to MCS.[1] According to the most recent community surveys, about 1.4% of the adult population suffers from panic disorders; the disorder also appears to be more common in women than in men. Recent evidence suggests that panic disorder results from dysregulation of central nervous system activity, in particular in the locus ceruleus (LC). In susceptible individuals, panic attacks may be provoked by lactate infusion peripherally, and extreme anxiety or panic may also be provoked by administration of centrally active substances that act to increase norepinephrine turnover in the LC and by substances that act as active antagonists to benzodiazepine receptors in the limbic system.[10] Minute exposures to some environmental chemicals might act directly on the central nervous system to cause panic attacks in some susceptible individuals (thus accounting for symptoms of MCS on a physiological basis). The large variety of chemicals that trigger symptoms in most individuals with the disorder make it unlikely that symptoms are caused by the direct action of chemicals on the brain. Rather, it seems more likely that cognitions and perceptions as well as chemicals cause anxiety and that errors in attribution account for the putative relationship between symptoms and chemical exposure in individuals with panic disorders or conditioned fear disorders.

Individuals with generalized anxiety disorders also suffer from a constellation of symptoms of autonomic hyperactivity, but because they experience symptoms continuously and for prolonged periods, rather than episodically as in panic disorder, their symptoms are less likely to be attributed to discrete exposures.

Individuals with post-traumatic stress disorder (PTSD) experience recurrent episodes of anxiety or panic (as well as diminished interest in activities, feelings of detachment from others, or constriction of affective responses) associated with the reexperiencing or recollection of a traumatic, life-threatening event. Schottenfeld and Cullen (1986) have recently described an atypical post-traumatic stress disorder, occurring most commonly in individuals who have been chronically exposed to noxious or toxic chemicals and who were terrified by symptoms and potential adverse health consequences of exposure.[22] In atypical PTSD, rather than recall the traumatic event in images or words, individuals reexperience the identical symptoms that were initially experienced at the time of exposure—these symptoms include a mixture of both irritant symptoms (caused by the direct effects of exposure on mucosal surfaces) and anxiety symptoms. As in typical PTSD, reexperiencing of symptoms in individuals with atypical PTSD is often caused by reminders of the initial traumatic event or by odors that resemble the initial exposure—eventually, a wide variety of odors may act as cues for evoking recurrent symptoms. Patients with atypical PTSD suffer from memories of their original, traumatic exposures, not from altered physiologic responses to exposure. Recognition that individuals can be harmed by the fear associated with an otherwise harmless exposure facilitates a diagnosis of atypical PTSD. Mrs. A., in this case history, suffered from both major depression and atypical PTSD.

CHEMICAL SENSITIVITIES AND SOMATOFORM DISORDERS

A somewhat confusing array of terms, including hysteria, conversion disorder, somatization disorder, Briquet's syndrome, and hypochondriasis have been used historically for the diagnosis of individuals suffering from an overlapping group of disorders currently referred to as somatoform disorders. In order to avoid confusion, in the discussion that follows I will adhere to the current diagnostic nosology formulated by the American Psychiatric Association. Many individuals considered to have MCS may in fact be suffering from one of the following somatoform disorders. Since these somatoform disorders were originally described prior to the introduction of many chemicals into the environment and often occur in the absence of chemical exposures, sensitivity to chemicals is not likely to account for the occurrence of these disorders.

A diagnosis of *hypochondriasis*, one discrete type of somatoform disorder, can be made for patients whose symptoms lead them to be preoccupied with the fear or belief of having a serious disorder, even in the absence of any physiological mechanism accounting for their symptoms and despite medical reassurance. A diagnosis of *conversion disorder* can be made for patients whose predominant disturbance is an involuntary loss or alteration in physical functioning that cannot be explained by any known physical disorder or pathophysiologic mechanism. The diagnostic hallmarks of *somatization disorder* are the occurrence of a large number (more than 14) of medically unexplained symptoms involving multiple organ systems—gastrointestinal, neurological, cardiorespiratory, genitourinary, and psychosexual symptoms—and onset prior to age 30. Somatization disorder is present in about 0.25% of the adult population in the United States and in 1% of adult women. Since patients with these disorders often insist on receiving overly extensive or invasive diagnostic procedures, unnecessary surgery, or harmful medical interventions, recognizing these disorders and limiting diagnostic, surgical, and medical interventions to the necessary minimum is essential to reduce the occurrence of iatrogenic complications. Patients who have a previous history of conversion symptoms (i.e., visual disturbances, difficulty in swallowing, fainting, memory loss, seizures, paralysis, aphonia, anesthesia, or coordination disturbance that occur without any neurological basis) and large numbers of other, medically unexplained, symptoms (such as shortness of breath, palpitations, chest pain, dizziness, abdominal discomfort, nausea, bloating, and dyspareunia) beginning before age 30 should receive a diagnosis of somatization disorder. Invoking a diagnosis of MCS in these patients is not likely to aid in caring for them and may actually lead to iatrogenic complications (e.g., social isolation and unnecessary restriction of activities).

IMPLICATIONS FOR PREVENTION AND TREATMENT

Consideration of the roles that cognitive processing, interpretive sets, emotional arousal and anxiety play in detection of chemical odors, symptom onset, and illness behavior suggests several interrelated intervention strategies for the prevention and treatment of MCS. Since the onset of symptoms of MCS often occurs in situations that are likely to lead individuals to be vigilant or alert to changes in their physical or somatic functioning (e.g., during times of organizational stress, labor-management disputes, and layoffs, or following frightening, potential or actual exposure to toxic substances), strategies that reduce stress are likely to reduce the incidence of the disorder and aid in recovery. Strategies that encourage greater participation of the employees in discovering and resolving potential workplace hazards may be particularly effective. Changes in the workplace that reduce toxic exposure and the risk of exposure may provide the most reassurance—the installation of a new exhaust system in Mrs. A.'s workplace was an extremely effective psychotherapeutic intervention in addition to its obvious benefit in the prevention of occupational respiratory disease.

Individuals who develop MCS often report that their symptoms were dismissed as trivial by their supervisors at work and by the health care personnel initially consulted. It should not be surprising that in situations of heightened suspicion these individuals have not been reassured that there was no cause for alarm about their symptoms. Since, to be effective, reassurance needs to come from trusted sources, even the most comprehensive and thorough evaluations conducted by company sponsored personnel may not be as reassuring as the opinion of health care experts chosen by the affected individual. Even when health information is provided by a trusted medical source, reassurance by dismissing symptoms as unimportant or inconsequential without providing sufficient information and knowledge to establish an alternative interpretive set for understanding symptoms and reducing anxiety is also likely to be ineffective. Further educational efforts must be directed at the entire affected "community" to be effective—many individuals who are not themselves symptomatic or ill may nevertheless support the mistaken interpretive set and illness behavior of the affected person. Finally, although secondary gains of illness may need to be reduced in order to alter the illness behavior of individuals with MCS, changes need to be made thoughtfully, carefully, and cautiously. Precipitously cutting off disability benefits or undermining family support are likely only to increase the anxiety of individuals with MCS and to exacerbate their symptoms. Medical practitioners need to chart a narrow course between an overly permissive stance that encourages excessive disability and an overly confrontational approach that exacerbates the illness of these patients. Although provision of sufficient and accurate information, caring, comfort and support are essential elements in the clinical management of individuals with MCS, a persistent insistence that the individual remain active in his or her social roles is also necessary to prevent regression into an overly dependent state and to prevent prolonged, excessive disability.

Specific cognitive and behavioral interventions may also be useful in the treatment of individuals with MCS. Desensitizing the individual (on a psychological rather than immunological basis) by gradually exposing the individual (at first in imagery and only later physically) to substances or situations associated with symptoms and teaching the individual to dampen symptoms by utilizing relaxation techniques or self-hypnosis may be one useful paradigm for treatment. Individuals with MCS may also be taught other cognitive techniques, such as directing attention away from symptoms or remembering that the symptoms are not indicative of life-threatening disease. The treatment of Mrs. A. utilized these cognitive and behavioral approaches, and it should be noted that Mrs. A. helped set the pace in the treatment. Training in biofeedback may also be useful in enabling the individual to learn techniques to modify bodily sensations. By providing the individual with an enhanced sense of control over symptoms, all of these techniques may also act to reduce the individual's anxiety about exposure and symptoms. The efficacy of the approach of clinical ecologists to the treatment of MCS may in fact result more from the unplanned and unintended psychological interventions of the clinical ecologist than from specific immunologic or nutritional manipulations.

Individuals with MCS will often need to learn and accept that complete cure or total relief from the occurrence of symptoms is not possible. Since symptoms of MCS are likely to reoccur, learning to accept and cope with recurrent symptoms is the optimal goal of successful treatment. Living on the hope of eventual cure (which will of necessity, at present, be unattainable) will eventuate in frustration, disappointment, and anger, and these emotional reactions will only complicate suffering and exacerbate disability. Clinicians involved in the treatment of individuals with MCS need to be cautious that their own therapeutic zeal and unrealistic hopes about effecting a cure do not contribute to the unrealistic expectations and ultimate disappointment of their patients.

Although it is not clear whether major depression or anxiety disorders are the cause of symptoms in individuals considered to have MCS, the result of the chronic illness experienced by these individuals, or a reflection of a common, underlying abnormality, treatment of these psychiatric disorders, when present, may often ameliorate symptoms and disability. Similar considerations hold for the treatment of post-traumatic stress disorders, which are also responsive to both pharmacologic and psychotherapeutic interventions. Both pharmacologic and psychotherapeutic interventions are effective in the treatment of major depression, anxiety, and post-traumatic stress disorders and are important adjuncts in the treatment of chemically sensitive individuals with these disorders. Although tricyclic antidepressant medications may be efficacious, many individuals with MCS appear to be unusually sensitive to the anticholinergic and sedative effects of this class of medications, and it is not always possible to achieve adequate therapeutic levels in these individuals. In addition to cognitive and behavioral psychotherapeutic techniques, which are discussed above and which are also efficacious in the treatment of these psychiatric disorders, interpersonal and supportive psychotherapies are also useful in the treatment of these disorders and may be of particular value in helping individuals with MCS learn to cope with their symptoms and disability, with the effects of the disorder on their relationships, and with the side effects of medications.

SUMMARY

Individuals considered to suffer from multiple chemical sensitivities comprise a heterogeneous grouping. Regardless of the original etiology of symptoms, these individuals tend to amplify their symptoms and to develop the mistaken belief that these symptoms are indicative of severe disease. Cognitive processes and anxiety contribute to amplification of symptoms and disability, and cognitive and behavioral techniques appear to be clinically useful in alleviating symptoms and disability. Specific psychiatric disorders, in particular major depression, panic disorder, post-traumatic stress disorder, and somatization disorder, may be confused or associated with MCS. When present, specific treatment of these psychiatric disorders is essential.

REFERENCES

1. American Psychiatric Association: Diagnostic and Statistical Manual of Mental Disorders, 3rd ed. Washington, DC, APA Press, 1980.
2. Astrachan BA, Price LR, Schottenfeld RS, Southwick SR: Psychiatric aspects of chronic pain. *In* Osterweis, M (ed): Pain and Disability: Clinical, Behavioral and Public Policy Perspectives. Washington, DC, National Academy Press (in press).
3. Barsky AJ and Klerman GL: Overview: Hypochondriasis, bodily complaints and somatic styles. Am J Psychiatry 140:273, 1983.
4. Brodsky CM: Psychological factors contributing to somatoform diseases attributed to the workplace. J Occup Med 25(6):459, 1983.
5. Bruch H: Anorexia nervosa: Therapy and theory. Am J Psychiatry 139(12):1531, 1981.
6. Cain W: (this issue).
7. Campbell D, Sanderson RE, Laverty SG: Characteristics of a conditioned reponse in human subjects during extinction trials following a single traumatic conditioning trial. J Abnorm Soc Psychol 68(6):627, 1964.
8. Detre TP, Jarecki HG: Modern Psychiatric Treatment. Philadelphia, JB Lippincott Co., 1971.
9. Eisenberg L: What makes persons "patients" and patients "Well" Am J Med 69:277, 1980.
10. Insel TR, Ninan PT, Aloi J, et al: A benzodiazepine receptor-mediated model of anxiety. Arch Gen Psychiatry 41:741, 1984.
11. Katon W, Ries RK, Kleinman A: The prevalence of somatization in primary care. Compr Psychiatry 25(2):208, 1984.
12. Kellner R: Functional somatic symptoms and hypochondriasis, A survey of empirical studies. Arch Gen Psychiatry 42:821, 1985.
13. Kessler LG, CLeary PD, Burke JD: Psychiatric disorders in primary care: Results of a follow-up study. Arch Gen Psychiatry 42:583, 1985.
14. National Center for Health Statistics: Selected Symptoms of Psychological Distress. Public Health Services Series 11, Number 37. Washington, DC, US Government Printing Office, 1970.
15. Pennebaker J, Skelton J: Psychological parameters of physical symptoms. Person Soc Psychol Bull 4:213, 1978.
16. Peterson WL, Sturdevant RAL, Frankl HD, et al: Healing of duodenal ulcer with an antacid regiman. N Engl J Med 297:341, 1977.
17. Regier DA, Myers JK, Kramer M, et al: The NIMH Epidemiologic Catchment Area Program. Arch Gen Psychiatry 41:934, 1984.
18. Regier DA, Goldberg ID, Taube CA: The DeFacto US Mental Health Service System: A public health perspective. Arch Gen Psychiatry 35:685, 1978.
19. Rodin J: Somatopsychics and attribution. Person Soc Psychol Bull 4:531, 1978.
20. Schacter S, Singer JE: Cognitive, social and psysiological determinants of emotional state. Psychol Rev 69:379, 1962.

21. Schottenfeld RS: Asbestos, lead and old lace: Psychiatric manifestations of toxic exposures in the workplace. Medical Times 142(2):198, 1985.
22. Schottenfeld RS, Cullen MR: Recognition of occupation-induced post-traumatic stress disorders. J Occup Med 28(5):365, 1986.
23. Shim C, William MH Jr: Effect of odors in asthma. Am J Med 80:18, 1986.
24. Skelton JA, Pennebaker JW: the psychology of physical symptoms and sensations. In Sanders GS, Suls J (eds): Social Psychology of Health and Illness. Hillsdale, New Jersey, Lawrence Erlbaum Associates.
25. Terr AI: Environmental illness—a clinical review of 50 cases. Arch Intern Med 146:145, 1986.

ROBERT K. McLELLAN, MD, MPH

BIOLOGICAL INTERVENTIONS IN THE TREATMENT OF PATIENTS WITH MULTIPLE CHEMICAL SENSITIVITIES

No more challenging clinical problem confronts the physician than treating the patient with multiple chemical sensitivities. The syndrome of multiple chemical sensitivities (MCS) is a chronic illness with many manifestations and probably multiple etiologies. General clinical management most appropriately resembles that for other chronic occupational diseases, such as chronic low back pain. Rarely are "cures" possible, though early intervention may hold such promise. Therapeutic goals should focus on decreasing social and physical disabilities by improving behavioral and physiologic coping behaviors and on assisting in the resolution of the often accompanying morass of psychosocial problems.

Satisfactory management of MCS demands Engel's psychobiosocial approach[41] and interdisciplinary cooperation among the helping professions. Although the emphasis of this presentation is on physiologic interventions, such biological approaches should only be applied in the context of a more holistic therapeutic strategem. Accordingly, although the details of psychosocial evaluation and management are left to authors of other disciplines, this paper is introduced by key philosophic and psychosocial considerations in the medical treatment of MCS.

The medical approaches described are eclectic. They do not represent the treatment model of either traditional clinical ecologists or occupational physicians. Most of the approaches described have been clinically applied by the author or his colleagues. Some have theoretical scientific merit, others have evolved empirically without a clear scientific rationale. In all cases, a profound lack of rigorous research prevents definitive statements about the general efficacy of described treatments. Instead, the author offers management techniques developed on the front line in the spirit of sharing clinical material that will hopefully provoke appropriate scientific study and that in the meantime will also provide clinicians with some therapeutic options.

THE SPECTRUM OF CHEMICAL SENSITIVITY

A wide spectrum of problems seem related to chemical sensitivity.* Such problems include several well-recognized syndromes, such as

---

From the Gesell Institute of Human Development New Haven, Connecticut

Reprint requests to Robert K. McLellan, MD, MPH, Gesell Institute of Human Development, 310 Prospect St., New Haven, CT 06511.

* The term sensitivity is used throughout this paper by convention. No immunologic meaning is implied. A better word at this point would be intolerance.

- isolated chemical sensitivities—toluene di-isocyanates;[17]
- sensitivity to a mix of very-low-level chemical exposures often found in indoor air pollution—tight building syndrome;[80]
- toxic effects of a single substance at very low levels of exposure because of poor host resistance related to such factors as concurrent disease,[129] age of patient[53] or diet;[22-23,45]
- epidemic illness falsely attributed to chemical exposure.[69]

This paper focuses on a sub-group of chemically sensitive patients that purposely excludes all of the above examples. The chief characteristics of this subgroup are

- **Symptoms on exposure to very low levels of chemicals**

The patient's symptoms occur on exposure to very low levels of chemicals (often at least an order of magnitude below commonly accepted hazardous levels). Symptoms are reportedly relieved by avoiding exposure to the offending chemicals. Note that patients without such relationships are excluded and that a currently unknown number of patients may believe in these relationships, where they may not actually be demonstrable. Difficulties in documenting the putative effects of low-level exposures have led to the span of medical opinion about the etiology of the symptoms reflected in this book.

- **Generalizing and increasing sensitivities**

Over time, the patient's symptoms are reportedly provoked by a smaller dose and a larger number of substances than initially was the case.[16,95,98,109] As a corollary, in my experience most MCS patients report symptoms on exposure not only to chemicals but also to a wide variety of other environmental exposures, e.g., respiratory allergens and foods. Because of this tendency, clinical ecologists have used the more inclusive term environmental illness (EI).

- **Multi-system, poly-symptomatic**

At the most extreme, patients may have a "positive review of symptoms," most of which are allegedly related to environmental intolerance. Clinical ecologists have in fact published papers attributing common medical problems as diverse as phlebitis and arthritis to EI.[98-100] The treatment approaches outlined here are centered on complaints related to the respiratory and ophthalmic mucosa and the central nervous system, because in this author's experience they are most common. Even in patients with symptoms related to many organ sytems, central neurologic and mucosal irritant complaints frequently stand out.

- **Complain more about their symptoms**

Doctors, lawyers, courts and workers' compensation commissions see a sub-group of MCS patients who complain about their symptoms. As with most other illnesses, it is probable that many people have symptoms on exposure to low levels of chemicals but do not complain or at least do not seek help.[68,146,151-152] A key factor that must be addressed in appropriate management of these patients is identifying the triggers that have prompted them to seek help.[130,152-153]

• **More disabled**

Not only does this subgroup of patients complain more about their symptoms but they are also more disabled by them.

TREATMENT PHILOSOPHY

The complexity of MCS requires a comprehensive, eclectic approach to meeting a patient's needs, many of which are not strictly medical. Multidisciplinary involvement is often necessary, but referral to other helping professionals such as social workers, psychotherapists and lawyers does not end the physician's responsibilities for creating an effective, holistic treatment plan. Key features that should play a role in such a plan are reviewed.

The chronicity of MCS[16,101,116] suggests that the physician should employ approaches that are useful in other chronic illnesses, such as diabetes or COPD. Since the hope for a "cure" is probably slim, rehabilitation and development of healthy coping behaviors should be emphasized. Realistic goal setting and timeliness for the achievement of these objectives figure importantly in treatment plans, e.g., participating in household chores by __, back to work by __, etc. Adoption of the sick role, appropriate for acute illness,[91] should be discouraged.[58-59] Maintaining or returning a sense of control to patients is important in treatment planning. MCS patients frequently identify themselves as victims. Such a posture may serve them well in courtrooms, workers' compensation hearings, or on soap boxes, calling for "detoxification" of our environment, but the identity as "victim" obstructs rehabilitation. Such insight has been an important part of the rehabilitation of incest victims who at a certain stage of their healing process are able to identify themselves as "survivors."[1] Similarly, a national group of formaldehyde-sensitive individuals recently changed their name from SUFFER (Save Us From Formaldehyde Environmental Repercussions) to CURE (Citizens United to Reduce Emissions of Formaldehyde Poisoning Association, Inc.). Referral to such self-help groups as CURE (Waconia, Minnesota 612-448-5441) for more information can introduce MCS patients to a supportive network of similarly afflicted people. Such groups, like those for other chronic illnesses, can serve as an important source of emotional support, as a clearinghouse of ideas for nonoffensive alternatives to common household chemicals, and as a grapevine for recommending understanding professionals. Unfortunately, at times these groups may obstruct rehabilitation by promoting coping behaviors that encourage isolation from mainstream society[16] and may abet psychophysiologic processes that lead to spreading and increasing sensitization. Psycho-educational groups with professional input may avoid some of the potentially counterproductive aspects of MCS groups but have the disadvantage of being professional rather than self-help sessions.[68] Family therapy or multi-family groups may prove critical in overcoming obstacles to rehabilitation created by family dynamics.

The doctor-patient relationship serves as an important tool in the treatment of MCS.[8] Because of the chronicity of MCS, effective therapeutic relationships are most likely going to be based on a partnership rather than an authoritarian model.[46,58,135] Careful listening to a patient's story can cement such a relationship. Acceptance and legitimization of a patient's concerns is crucial to successful on-going communication.[14]

No more sensitive issue permeates the doctor-patient relationship than the relative importance of mind and body in the pathophysiology of MCS. Commonly an MCS patient's complaints have been disbelieved by employers, friends or family or have been labelled as "all in you head."[97] Adjectives, perceived as derogatory, such as "hysterical" or "somatisizing," have been used to describe their symptoms. In turn, these patients frequently feel as though no one "believes" them. They become resistant to acknowledging the importance of psychosocial components of their illness. Furthermore, clinical ecology has promoted physiological explanations for a wide spectrum of symptoms and at the same time disparaged psychological explanations.[97] Treatment must begin with a discussion of contributory psychosocial as well as physiologic factors. Yet, the clinician must show sensitivity to the central need these patients have for a vindication of an environmental basis for their symptoms. To deny this basis outright may quickly alienate the patient and also be wrong. Not understanding the physiologic mechanisms cannot excuse thorough investigation of the patient's theories. As with many other chronic illnesses, MS patients have much to teach their care providers.

The language used by the physician can critically affect the patient's rehabilitation. Diagnostic labels such as MCS or environmental illness can have tremendous therapeutic benefit ("At last I know what I have!"),[137] but mislabelling is always a risk. Parsimonious psychological or physiological diagnoses may obstruct thorough investigation of all contributing factors. As worrisome are the use of quasi-diagnostic labels, such as "pan-allergic" or "allergic to the 20th century disease."[54] Such terms can only add to disabling psychophysiologic burdens carried by MCS patients.[81] Problem lists, as encouraged by Weed,[145] including complaints, laboratory abnormalities, as well as diagnoses, are suggested as an aid in avoiding the constructions of simplistic labels.

Difficult patient relational styles are common. Anger, though not always overtly expressed, is one common theme. Patients are angry at doctors who have not believed them, who have told them that there was nothing wrong with them, and who have given them drugs that have made them feel worse. MCS patients are often angry at other authorities—employers, manufacturers, and other perceived perpetrators of environmental illness. Compulsive adherence to professionally or self-prescribed lifestyle restrictions creates problems with all social contacts, including with health care providers. Some MCS patients are spectacularly well-informed about the chemical ingredients of virtually everything. Learn from these people without defensiveness. Within reason, accommodate to requests for additive-free medications, an office where staff does not wear perfume, etc. On the other hand, limit-setting is crucial to a lasting therapeutic relationship. Just as part of MCS patients' illness is the degree to which their lives revolve around their illness, so they may overwhelm their doctors with endless questions, lists of symptoms, and requests that special environmental accommodations be made for them.

No matter what their medical problem, the ultimate event that triggers most patients to seek medical care is psychosocial.[152] Unless this need is elicited, the patient may well leave the doctor's office unsatisfied.[150] As with other patients, the underlying cause for seeking medical care may not be discovered except through deliberate and persistent attention to the patients unconscious as well as conscious behavior.

Frequently, the MCS patient presents with at least some clearly identified social needs that require medical input. These include documentation of a patient's eligibility for various social benefits, such as workers' compensation or social security disability. As well, the physician may be asked to encourage employers and families to modify work and living environments. Financial set-backs incurred through job loss and modification of homes may prompt patients to ask doctors to supply medical justification for loan forgiveness, etc. In attending to these social needs, the physician not only must judge the medical worthiness of the patient's claims but also must consider the overall therapeutic value of encouraging such patient endeavors. On one hand, involvement in compensation hearings and litigation may prove to be a healthy and legitimate focus for anger that would otherwise obstruct rehabilitation. On the other hand, all too often the litigation process is not only demeaning but also lengthy and may itself become a factor in delaying rehabilitation.[9,83,138] Part of a physician's responsibility in participating in litigation, or in documenting disability, must be to alert the patient to the potentially "sickening" aspects of social benefit programs and litigation.

Diagnostic procedures as described by other authors in this issue will help clarify the relative importance of physiological and psychological interventions, but rarely are both not necessary. Psychophysiologic explanations of the concepts of conditioned responses and post-traumatic stress disorder[116] are helpful in gaining patient acceptance of psychological interventions.

In deciding to refer a MCS patient for psychotherapy, many of the same criteria useful in the management of other chronic illnesses are helpful. These criteria include:

- disability far out of proportion to measurable physiological impairment;
- significant family dysfunction as can be quickly assessed by such measures as the family APGAR;[122]
- fixation at an early developmental aspect of the illness, i.e., at a stage of helplessness, anger and victimization;
- concurrent psychopathology that usually warrants referral, e.g., serious depression, psychotic disorders, and the special case of post-traumatic stress disorder.

BIOLOGICAL INTERVENTIONS

Two questions should frame the clinician's therapeutic plan for the chemically sensitive patient. What is the patient sensitive to and why is he or she so sensitive? The answer to the first question is used to design a program of avoidance that will reduce symptoms. Investigating the second point is both more challenging and potentially more rewarding. This author's experience, along with others', [6,20] suggests that MCS patients often go to extremes to avoid common low-dose chemical exposures, leading to social isolation and sometimes complete disability from work. Thus, notwithstanding the value of avoidance, the primary goal of treatment must be to decrease sensitivities.

WHAT IS THE PATIENT SENSITIVE TO?

A careful medical, environmental, and occupational history will elicit the onset and recurrent precipitation of symptoms by certain exposures. In contrast to the picture in a worker with a specific sensitivity, the history of the MCS patient will (by definition) reveal broad classes of putative offensive agents. Despite controversy[3,136] about validity, reliability, and significance, sublingual and intradermal provocative challenge,[36,47,61] antibody[92,147] testing, and direct biological assay[102] for specific substances have been used to direct attention to groups of agents, e.g., organic solvents, pesticides, or gaseous irritants. Refinement of immunologic techniques[92,147] and inhalation provocation with objective dependent variables as reported by Gyntelberg[50] show promise of being useful techniques for determining what chemicals a patient should avoid.

Two key hypotheses of clinical ecology are relevant to an avoidance program. The first is the concept of "total environmental load" (TEL). This idea corresponds to the traditional toxicological concept of "total industrial hygiene load." The TEL expands the toxicological precept that knowledge of the sum of all toxic exposures to an individual is key to predicting health effects. TEL goes beyond the environment of toxins to include all potential stressors, particularly food intolerances, common inhalant allergies, and psychosocial stresses.[12] The concept further suggests that symptoms occur when the individual's capacity for coping with the varied stresses is overwhelmed. In theory, reducing the TEL will decrease an individual's sensitivities to any given substance. Immunologists have objected to this thesis because, given the specificity of the immune system and the lack of supportive evidence, there is little reason to believe in the soundness of the hypothesis.[3] Much of the conflict, however, has resulted because of different uses of the word allergy or sensitivity. Although some of the effects of low-dose chemical exposures on the MCS patient may be immunologically mediated, many may not be. Thus, in the most global sense there probably can be agreement that the sum of a variety of factors may depress and/or overwhelm an organism's coping capacity.[2] More specifically, for example, during the stress of rotating shift work, an individual is likely to be more sensitive to the toxic effects of a variety of substances.[75] Or, a viral gastroenteritis will result in an increase in lactose intolerance.[124] Or, an asthmatic allergic to ragweed will be less tolerant of a gaseous irritant during ragweed season.[45] The therapeutic implications of TEL are that avoidance of a variety of potential environmental stressors may decrease a person's symptoms on exposure to any given chemical.

Immunologic cross-reactivity between foods, chemicals and common inhalant allergens may add to the importance of TEL. Although little rigorous documentation of such cross-reactivity exists, some surprising examples have been reported that warrant further exploration of the more general hypothesis.[21] Some clinical ecology pioneers have suggested that very general chemical classes, e.g., "petrochemicals," may all affect a MCS patient because of chemical similarities that result in cross-reactivity.[95] Other authors have speculated that such reactions may extend to the wide variety of phenyl compounds naturally occurring in food and therefore explain the phenomenon of multiple food intolerances coexisting with MCS.[79]

The second key hypothesis advanced by clinical ecology stems from the clinical observation that chronic symptoms in some patients may be the result of imperfect physiologic adaptation to on-going low-level chemical exposures.[95] The temporal relationship between symptoms and exposures is masked until "total chemical avoidance" is achieved. Theoretically, over time (usually days) the chronic symptoms disappear. (Such "total avoidance" is achieved in environmental units built with "non-toxic" materials and supplied with carefully purified air.) Total avoidance "unmasks" symptom/exposure relationships so that either purposeful (in the environmental unit) or incidental (in the real world) reexposure results in *acute* symptoms. In other words, in effect the patient becomes "more sensitive" after brief total avoidance. According to this theory, prolonged avoidance, over weeks or months, will result in decreasing sensitivity and renewed "tolerance." Future *repeated* exposures run the risk of recreating the masked state of chronic symptoms. This theory is an extension of Rinkel's[107] concept of chronic food allergy. Although many descriptive case histories supportive of Randolph's theory exist in the literature,[36,95,98–101] rigorous documentation is lacking. On the other hand, enough related pieces of physiology and toxicology are supportive of a general notion such as Randolph's that further inquiry into its validity is warranted.

In this author's experience, a program of environmental avoidance works most satisfactorily for people whose symptoms are limited to mucosal irritation. Avoidance is most troublesome for people who have more pervasive symptoms. These patients are characterized by relentlessly increasing and generalizing sensitivities that lead to severely restricted lifestyles. If this process is observed, recommendations for global environmental restrictions are likely to result only in greater isolation and disability.

In general, the design and rationale for an avoidance program resembles recommendations made for people with standard respiratory allergies. The home, in particular the bedroom, should serve as an oasis from suspected offensive environmental agents. Nonoffensive alternatives should be substituted for incriminated household sources of indoor air pollution. Several practical reviews of measures to correct indoor air pollution exist.[26,51,67,85,95] Corrective measures include consideration of occupants' habits (e.g., smoking), hobbies (e.g., furniture refinishing), appliances (e.g., unvented kerosene heaters), furnishings (e.g., particleboard furniture), household products (e.g., formaldehyde-based air purifiers), and cosmetics (e.g., formaldehyde-based shampoos). Occasionally, the actual structure of the home and its ventilation deserves manipulation. For example, if airborne levels of formaldehyde are significant in a dwelling insulated with urea formaldehyde, foam removal can effectively lower these levels, though at great expense.[121]

As an alternative to product substitution, improved ventilation or air purification may be appropriate. Tightly built new homes with little fresh air infiltration may have ventilation increased with heat exchangers with little loss of energy efficiency. Other individuals may benefit from portable air purifiers (a model that can be installed in a car is also available[32]).

Humidification plays a major role in mediating the health impact of airborne irritants. Increasing humidity decreases irritant symptoms, but as relative humidity increases beyond 50%, problems arise: microbial growth (especially molds) is encouraged; structural damage to the living space may occur; and hydrolysis of formaldehyde resins may increase formaldehyde off-gassing. Ideal indoor relative humidity in winter is probably between 40–50%,[4,90] though very low outdoor temperatures may lower these figures. Special attention must be paid to regular cleaning of portable or central humidifiers to control microbial growth.

Although MCS patients obviously have less control over their work environment, the physician should assist them in requesting reasonable modifications such as provision of a nonsmoking work place, proper humidification and appropriate ventilation.[80,127–128]

A MCS patient's chemical environment includes food, water, and medications. Again, with the notion that decreasing an individual's TEL may be theoretically beneficial, attention to eating and drinking substances free of potentially offending chemicals may be indicated.[95] A healthy, whole food diet is prescribed, preferably free of intentional and unintentional chemical additives. Similarly, good drinking water is recommended. An alarming number of private wells are contaminated with a wide variety of toxic substances.[6,60,62] Public water supplies are monitored for only a fraction of possible chemical contaminants[60] and are usually treated with chlorine or chlorine dioxide, substances that chemically sensitive people may be troubled by.[28,126] When an alternative source of water is indicated based on water analysis or based on symptoms provoked by double-blind challenges with tap water versus "pure" water, this author generally recommends household water purification rather than bottled water. There are two rationales for this recommendation. First, bottled water is less regulated than public water supplies. Some local bottled water vendors have been cited for distributing microbiologically contaminated water or water with unsafe levels of minerals.[35,52,60] In addition, if water is purchased in soft plastic containers, the MCS patient may be intolerant of trace plastic leachates in the water. The second reason for suggesting point-of-use water purification is that research has suggested that approximately 70% of an individual's daily absorbed dose of volatile organic chemicals is from bathing water.[19] As well, the irritant effects of aerosolized and vaporized chlorine may be intolerable for some MCS patients. Therefore, if water is an issue, decontaminated bathing water may be an even higher priority than purified drinking water. A variety of water purification systems is available, some of which may compound rather than solve a problem of water impurity.[60,144]

MCS patients are also frequently intolerant of a wide variety of medications. The use of any medication should of course be minimized. If medications are indicated, those that are free of unnecessary chemical additives (such as colors and flavors) should be prescribed. A list of additive free drugs is available from The Feingold Association of the United States (PO Box 6550, Alexandria, VA 22306). Lifestyle drugs such as ethanol, tobacco, and caffeine are also usually best avoided.

Some MCS patients go to extreme lengths to avoid chemical exposures. One such measure includes the use of gas masks equipped with a variety of filters. Although such measures seem bizarre and counterproductive, this author cared for one MCS patient whose use of a mask was adaptive. She suffered from such severe bronchial hyperreactivity that when exposed to low levels of airborne irritants she frequently (4 times a year) went into true respiratory arrest requiring resuscitation and mechanical ventilatory assistance. This patient used a mask to maintain a semblance of a normal lifestyle, continuing to do her own household errands. Similarly, allergists frequently prescribe pollen masks for respiratory allergy sufferers when they are involved in such activities as lawn cutting, gardening or house cleaning.

To a degree, the kind of environmental manipulations described are sensible for anyone with the reasonable desire to reduce unnecessary exposures to potentially toxic substances. When taken to an extreme, such interventions can be both financially and emotionally exhausting, particularly for a family with a chronically ill member. As well, finding non-toxic alternatives may not always be easy. For this reason, the physician should consider referring a MCS patient to a support network such as HEAL (Human Ecology Action League, 7330 North Rogers Ave, Chicago, IL 60626) or CURE (Waconia, MN 55387–9583). Some national newsletters also serve as a support system.[42,108] Local unaffiliated support groups also often exist. Comprehensive catalogues of household supplies for the chemically sensitive allow mail-order shopping for items that range from organic food to pure cotton clothes to cosmetics and housewares.[31]

Aside from the economic, social, and psychological dislocations involved in the more extreme cases of environmental avoidance, there is a very real danger that such manipulations may actually make problems worse. Clinically, such apparent aggravation of problems is not uncommon. There are two theoretical reasons for this. First, to the extent that the phenomenon of chemical sensitivity is a conditioned behavior, MCS patients may be taught to be even more sensitive by the well-meaning attentions of clinicians and support groups who suggest environmental avoidance. Second, some degree of chemical exposures may be important in inducing detoxification enzymes that protect against deleterious physiological responses to low levels of chemicals. The unavoidable, inadvertent exposure may thus trigger an unusually strong response in the "chemically naive" person. Well-understood examples of this exist. For example, the teetotaler is more easily inebriated than someone who has a two-beer-a-day habit. Particularly relevant is the fact that olfactory fatigue occurs on continued exposure to a specific substance; avoidance of the substance allows greatly increased olfactory sensitivity.[84]

To summarize, chemical avoidance can play an important role in decreasing the symptoms of a MCS patient. There is good precedent for the helpfulness of environmental manipulation when traditional allergy or toxicology is considered. Many chemical exposures may be reduced by measures that are sensible for all of us and may be generally beneficial. Further reductions in exposures can be designed based on a person's specific intolerances and the severity of these intolerances. Extreme caution, however, must be exercised in suggesting drastic environmental regimens to avoid iatrogenically increasing the patient's sensitivities and disabilities. Judgments about the degree of recommended restriction are based on such issues as psychosocial hardships created by lifestyle changes and on clinical response to this type of management. Particular care should be used in recommending measures that will clearly identify the patient as "sick," e.g., a gas mask. The main goal of treatment should be maintaining sensible, healthy lifestyles by improving tolerance rather than using extremes of environmental avoidance.

FIRST AID

Several first-aid measures have been proposed by clinical ecologists for the management of MCS patients' acute reaction to low levels of chemicals. One group of these methods is based on standard treatment of acute poisoning. The other group has evolved clinically and generally remains to be rigorously evaluated.

First aid for the acute reaction of the MCS individual involves steps to stop the chemical's absorption. Most simply, the patient should leave the contaminated environment, terminate ingestion of the suspected food, or interrupt contact with the offending agent. Depending on the severity of the reaction, the next step involves decontamination through skin washing with soap and water, eye irrigation with sterile saline, or a variety of gastrointestinal interventions. Such interventions may include the induction of vomiting, the use of activated charcoal, and/or the use of a purgative.[12] Randolph[95] has indicated that the administration of 100% oxygen for several minutes or of intravenous sodium bicarbonate can abort a chemical sensitivity reaction. He rationalizes this therapy with the theory that hypoxia and lactic acidosis are important intermediaries in the MCS patients' adverse responses to environmental agents.[96]

The other group of immediate treatment methods that has been advocated includes oral alkali salts (sodium and potassium bicarbonate in a 2:1 ratio; commercially available as Alka-Seltzer without aspirin), sublingual drops of heparin adrenalin, and oral or intravenous pyridoxine and/or vitamin C.[93,125] If used judiciously, it is unlikely that any of these is harmful. On the other hand, at this point their efficacy has not been rigorously evaluated. The use of ophthalmic wetting drops and nasal mucosal lubrication with water-soluble jellies (avoiding petroleum jelly) clearly has a place in the symptomatic treatment of patients with mucosal irritation.

WHY IS THE PATIENT SO SENSITIVE?

Biological Interventions to Improve Tolerance

Toxicology recognizes inter- and intraspecies variability of response to specific toxins. Some factors that modulate the differences are immutable e.g., species, sex, and age. Other factors have been identified from animal experiments that may both modify an organism's response to a toxic agent and be amenable to manipulation. Several such variables have been explored in research with human subjects and are relevant to improving the tolerance of chemically sensitive patients. Other measures currently in vogue among clinical ecologists for treating MCS patients have less justification but merit evaluation.

INTERCURRENT DISEASE

Strong justification exists to suggest that intercurrent pathophysiologic alterations may alter the sensitivity of a human to a chemical.[45] One example is the relative intolerance of a patient with angina to carbon monoxide.[44] Perhaps more relevant, asthmatics or individuals with allergic rhinitis are much more intolerant of certain chemical irritants than a well population.[34] Appropriate treatment of underlying conditions may improve a patient's chemical tolerance. Treatment of the MCS patient requires not only optimal management of known illnesses but also appropriate investigation for possibly relevant, undiscovered problems.

The possibility of typical respiratory allergy and food intolerance deserves special attention. MCS patients with complaints of rhinitis, conjunctivitis, pharyngitis, sinusitis, and asthma should be thoroughly evaluated for the possibility of atopy. Not only is it clear that people with allergic mucosa are often more sensitive to irritants, mucosal irritation by viral or irritant exposures may themselves set the stage for sensitization with common allergens.[10,40,65,89,134] People may be exposed to irritants and airborne allergens simultaneously. For example, urea formaldehyde foam insulation has been found to be an excellent media for mold growth.[43] If atopy is confirmed, the MCS patient whose chief complaints relate to the respiratory and ophthalmic mucosa may be significantly helped by such measures as environmental interventions to decrease exposure to offending allergens (cats, molds, dust mites, etc.), allergy medications and immunotherapy.

Clinical ecologists consider evaluation and treatment for food intolerance an integral part of the treatment of MCS patients. Aside from the issue of potential intolerance to food additives, various other attributes of food and the digestive process are considered possible contributors to the MCS syndrome, particularly when neuropsychiatric symptoms are paramount. Bell[12] has reviewed several non-reaginic mechanisms postulated as triggers of such symptoms. These hypotheses include:

1. Foods supply neurotransmitter precursors that can affect brain levels of neurotransmitters and thereby behavior and emotions.

2. Digestion generates pharmacologically active agents such as opioid peptides that may cross the blood-brain barrier.

3. Digestive hormones and the activation of other hormones by food in the gut may impact on central neural activity.

4. Immune complexes formed by food antigens may alter the blood-brain barrier and thereby lead to CNS aberrations.

5. During digestion, particular foods may stimulate intestinal-neural signals and vice versa, especially to the hypothalamus, that specify particular behaviors and feelings.

6. The volatile chemicals of food odors stimulate olfactory-limbic system pathways, resulting in adverse reactions to specific foods. Such pathways may be similarly stimulated by low-level environmental chemical exposures, resulting in the observed patterns of multiple sensitivities and cross-reactivities.

Treatment of food intolerance involves most simply avoidance of offending foods. Without rigorous justification, clinical ecologists often recommend a "rotary diversified" diet, rather than or in addition to elimination diets, on the theory that food intolerance is created and exacerbated by monotonous diets that result in frequent ingestion of the same foods.[97] Golos[49] thoroughly describes how to design a rotary diet. Such diets can demand fanatical meal planning and in this author's experience carry the same psychosocial risks as extreme environmental avoidance. On the other hand, a modified rotary diet that includes a wide range of foods may be much preferable to the severely restricted menu that the sickest MCS patients limit themselves to. Several other controversial methods of managing food intolerances have been used, e.g., immunotherapy, digestive aids, and "neutralization" of presumably immunologic reactions to naturally occurring phenyl compounds in foods.[12]

Unfortunately, treatment of intercurrent illnesses may compound the problem of MCS. Aside from their desired effects in the management of a specific problem, medications may induce enzymes that theoretically could increase a patient's tolerance of certain chemicals. There is little scientific evidence that supports this use of medications to alleviate MCS. On the other hand, prescribed drugs do frequently exacerbate MCS. Possible mechanisms include specific target-organ actions, the presence of potentially troublesome ingredients, interactions of drugs with absorbed chemicals, and drug-related nutritional depletion. For example, decongestants may dry nasal mucosa and make it more susceptible to irritant injury. Or antiinflammatory drugs may disrupt intestinal mucosal integrity and allow increased absorption of food antigens and contaminants. Sulfites in inhaled bronchodilators may exacerbate asthma in sulfite intolerant individuals.[132] Alpha-adrenergic stimulants in decongestants may increase susceptibility to arrhythmias on exposure to halogenated hydrocarbons.[111] Diuretics may lead to potassium and magnesium depletion, resulting in increased neuromuscular irritability. In sum, medications should be used sparingly in MCS patients and, as mentioned previously, should be additive free if possible. Paring down a MCS patients pharmaceutical burden may increase tolerance to other chemicals.

CHRONOBIOLOGY

Variations in the chemical tolerance of organisms are certainly related to chronobiological factors.[27,38,75] Luce[75] reviews the circadian toxicity rhythms of a number of substances such as anesthetics, nicotine, strychnine, salicylates and others. Similarly, Reinberg[104,105] has documented rhythmically changing skin wheals of allergic subjects. Healthy individuals were found to have similar cyclic changes in their response to intradermal histamine.

Dysynchronicity refers to a disturbance in the normal relationships of the variety of cyclic body rhythms such as diurnal hormonal swings, temperature fluctuation, metabolic changes and excretion patterns. Many biological rhythms are easily measured and their normal patterns are well described.[75] Dysynchronicity can thus be easily identified. Causes of dysynchronicity include jet travel across time zones, rotating shift work, sleep disturbances (both a cause and symptom of dysynchronicity), drugs such as methylxanthines, including both caffeine and theophylline preparations, and chronic illness.[106] Theoretically, chronic dysynchronicity is common and evidence suggests that it decreases an organism's tolerance to a variety of stressors.[75] Correction of this chronobiological disorder may be valuable in improving the chemical tolerance of a MCS patient. For example, Karnovsky[57] has reviewed recent progress in sleep research that draws connections between the immune system and sleep disorders. Ehret[39] has described a simple plan for improving "chronohygiene" that involves manipulation of a variety of Zeitgebers (biological time setters), including dietary modifications, pharmacologic agents and exercise.

NUTRITIONAL INTERVENTIONS

There is little doubt that an organism's nutritional status plays an important role in determining its response to certain chemical exposures.[22,23,38] As Galland has indicated earlier in this volume, a wide range of nutritional disturbances is commonly discovered in MCS patients. Whether these problems are the result of the illness or behavior associated with MCS or predate the syndrome is unknown. In either case nutritional disorders may compound MCS. Use of nutrients in pharmacologic doses may improve patients' chemical tolerance and overall well being.

Calabrese[22,23] has extensively reviewed the interaction of nutritional status with toxic response. Several factors must be considered before over-enthusiastically applying knowledge about such interactions:

1. There is a dearth of human data.

2. Most research focuses on the interactions of single nutrients with single toxins in high doses, whereas the nature of MCS is that the individual is usually intolerant to a wide variety of substances at much lower doses.

3. The pathophysiology of MCS may be different than that occurring with the high-dose exposures usually studied, e.g., CNS syndromes may be based on olfactory-limbic links with little relevance to hepatic metabolism.[15,64,148]

On the other hand:

1. The nutritional status of an individual can be readily ascertained.

2. Within reason, nutritional manipulations can be made safely.

3. Extant literature does provide theoretical support for the therapeutic use of nutritional management, especially as it related to the MCS patients with symptoms of mucosal irritation. And, nutrient abnormalities, such as B vitamin deficiencies may, themselves be responsible for some of the neurologic symptoms found with many MCS patients.

Therefore, a thorough nutritional status evaluation is indicated for any chronically ill individual with MCS. Such investigation should include not only a dietary history and a physical exam but also the range of biochemical studies as outlined by Dr. Galland. Based on the results of a comprehensive nutritional survey, appropriate recommendations may be made for dietary changes and supplementation with replacement doses of specific nutrients.

A general biochemical theory of chemical sensitivity has been proposed by Levine.[70] In essence, he suggests that sensitivity occurs as normal antioxidant defenses are overwhelmed either by exposure to exogenous oxidizing chemicals or through infection that stimulates phagocytic production of free radicals. Additionally, other authors point out that free radical production may trigger inflammatory prostaglandin synthesis.[82] Levine[70] also notes that numerous representatives of the chemical classes that cause chemical sensitivity reactions (e.g., aromatic hydrocarbons, chlorinated hydrocarbons, or the photochemical oxidants) exist either as free radicals in the aqueous tissue environment or are capable of being metabolized to free-radical intermediates by cellular xenobiotic enzymes, such as cytochrome P450 oxidase, aryl hydrocarbon hydroxylase, or a wide variety of metabolic oxidoreductases. If Levine's theory is correct, supplementing a MCS patient with antioxidant nutrients and/or inhibiting with prostaglandin synthesis should be helpful.

Some data exists to suggest that the oxidant/prostaglandin theory of chemical intolerance is at least partially valid. First, in this book Galland has outlined a pattern of nutritional abnormalities that suggests antioxidant depletion in MCS patients, e.g., low plasma selenium, abnormal erythrocyte superoxidase dismutase (a copper dependent enzyme), abnormal erythrocyte glutathione peroxidase (a selenium-dependent enzyme), and fatty acid metabolic disorders, which may lead to disruptions in normal prostaglandin synthesis. Second, although surprisingly scanty and by no means conclusive, both animal and human research have supported the notion that supplementation with antioxidants such as selenium, Vitamin C, the retenoids, some B vitamins, and the tocopherols may be helpful in protection against the toxicity of such irritant gases as ozone, sulfur dioxide, and nitrogen dioxide.[22–23,25,30,37–38] Other antioxidants such as the amino acids methionine and dimethyl glycine may also theoretically be of benefit.[25,70] Third, vitamin E has been shown to have antiinflammatory properties, with some of this effect explained by its impact on prostaglandin synthesis.[71]

Measurement of lipid peroxides, essential fatty acid metabolites and indices of antioxidant depletion may prove useful in decisions to use nutritional supplementation in the treatment of MCS patients. Pharmacological doses of these nutrients may have a protective antioxidant effect beyond replacement of deficiencies. Furthermore, toxicity mechanisms other than oxidation may respond to nutrient supplementation.[22-23] Manipulation of dietary fatty acids may prove useful both in affecting beneficially cell membrane structure as well as in inhibiting inflammatory prostaglandin synthesis.[103,113]

In sum, the author includes nutritional interventions in the care of virtually all of his MCS patients. The initial emphasis is on ensuring a balanced high-fiber diet that minimizes intake of synthetic chemicals and on replacing specific nutrients found deficient in physical and laboratory examination. Subsequently, a therapeutic trial of a mixed antioxidant nutritional supplement such as Anti-Ox (Allergy Research Group) is tried. Dietary fats are manipulated to decrease total fat intake to about 30% of calories, with an equal division between saturated, cold-pressed, nonhydrogenated polyunsaturated, and monounsaturated fats. If fat is used in cooking, saturated and monounsaturated fats are recommended. This plan effectively decreases the possible oxidant load from fat and minimizes possible fatty acid metabolic disturbances resulting from a diet high in saturated fats and/or the common trans, partially hydrogenated fats present in margarine and many processed foods.[113] If fatty acid metabolites are not measured, therapeutic trials for a month of gamma-linolenic acid [available as Effamol {Murdock Pharmaceuticals, Inc.}, 3 capsules twice a day] or eicosopentanoeic acid [such as Maxepa {STUR DEE}, 4 capsules twice a day] may be used in mucosal irritant syndromes as an attempt to decrease inflammatory prostaglandins and improve tissue integrity with little risk of significant adverse effects.

PSYCHOPHYSIOLOGIC INTERVENTIONS

The techniques of behavioral medicine hold great promise for the treatment of MCS. An enormous literature supports the notion that psychophysiologic intervention may prove useful in modifying illness, whatever pathologic mechanism may be involved in MCS.[73-74]

To the extent that symptoms of MCS are learned behaviors, a possible approach to treatment would involve deconditioning. During purposeful exposure to low doses of offensive chemicals, pathophysiologic responses could be interrupted by a variety of techniques designed to evoke the relaxation response.[13,33,117]

Alternatively, advantage may be taken of the olfactory-limbic theory by blocking adverse reactions to offensive odors with the administration of fragrances perceived by the subject as pleasant. Neurophysiologic data suggests that different odors stimulate distinctive cerebral electrophysiologic patterns[64]; some indicate an alerting response and others a relaxation response. Such patterns in combination with a subject's report could be used to pick a specific odor to be employed as needed to abort reactions to offensive chemicals. Schwartz has successfully used this technique in preventing and interrupting cataleptic responses in a complicated MCS patient.[118] A variety of odors produced by low-level chemical exposures (not involving known antigens) have been shown to precipitate asthma and nasal symptoms.[18,120] Regardless of the mechanism for this response, theoretically other odors may be effective in relieving symptoms. In fact, an ancient healing art known as aromatherapy, much practiced in Europe, has begun to gain popularity in the United States and promotes remedies that warrant investigation for the alleviation of the respiratory maladies of MCS.[143]

MICROBIOLOGICAL DISRUPTIONS

A highly speculative theory for treatment of the MCS syndrome proposes interventions to correct observed disturbances of a person's normal microbial ecology. In brief, clinicians caring for chemically sensitive patients have often noted associated symptoms, signs, and laboratory data that suggest chronic or frequent infections or more subtle changes in these patients' normal microbial flora.[7,139] Although there has been no rigorous attempt to ascertain the prevalence of these associations, a relevant research literature exists.

Most published, clinical discussions of this theory have focussed on the impact of *Candida albicans* on its host.[70,140–142] A MCS patient with an associated problem with Candida often presents as follows: chronic upper respiratory infections occurring in the setting of initially often unrecognized exposure to airborne irritants are treated repetitively with antibiotics over a course of months to years. Overt oropharyngeal, vaginal, or intestinal candidiasis becomes a recurrent problem as the patient's chemical sensitivities intensify. Laboratory findings implicating a Candida problem may include culture and microscopic identification, and the presence of immediate hypersensitivity or the absence of delayed hypersensitivity on skin testing with Candida antigen, abnormal IgA, IgM, IgG, or IgE serum Candida antibodies.[5,77,78,110,119,123,140–142]

Candidiasis may merely be an epiphenomenon of MCS, but several theories have evolved that explain how Candidiasis may contribute to chemical intolerance:

1. Candida infection decreases mucosal integrity, thereby enhancing susceptibility to chemical irritation or sensitization. (Intestinal dysbacteriosis has been cited as a factor in the sensitization to foods.[66])
2. Abundant Candida colonization may be sufficient to create immunological abnormalities.[48,70,77]
3. Candida may elaborate mycotoxins that add to the toxicity of chemical exposures.[24,29,56,139]
4. Chronic candidiasis may stimulate phagocytes to produce excess oxidants that overburden the body's antioxidant buffering capacity and lead to decreased chemical tolerance.[70]

For those patients with MCS and evidence of chronic candidiasis, treatment of the Candida problem may bring some relief of the MCS syndrome. Fully described by Truss,[140] the regimen usually involves dietary modification (a decrease in simple sugars and yeast and mold foods), prolonged oral nystatin along with topical nystatin when appropriate, and sometimes immunotherapy with the Candida antigen.

DETOXIFICATION

Xenobiotic chemical burdens may contribute to an individual's intolerance of additional chemical exposures in a variety of ways, e.g., by genetic, metabolic, or immunologic effects. Organohalides have received particular attention because they are lipophilic, have very long biological half-lives, and pose a broad exposure threat. They have been found to be ubiquitous contaminants in human tissues.[87,114] As a class, they tend to be potent inducers of various enzyme systems, including mixed function oxidases relevant to the metabolism of other xenobiotics. Chronic toxicities of heavy exposures are legion and include neurologic, metabolic, and possibly immunologic abnormalities relevant to MCS.[11,55,76,88,94,102]

If there is a relationship between chemical intolerance and low-level xenobiotic burden, a means of reducing this burden could be an important management tool. Several attempts have been made.[72,112,115,131] One approach has been found safe and efficacious by Schnare in a pilot trial with seven human subjects.[114] The treatment is an approximately three-week regimen of polyunsaturated oil supplement, aerobic exercise, sauna at 60–82 F, supplements of vitamins and minerals centered around nicotinic acid, water and salts to avert electrolyte imbalances due to sweating, and a regimented daily schedule with balanced meals and adequate sleep. Concern persists however that such regimens may result in acute toxicities as stored toxins are liberated into the blood stream.[63] As well, unfortunately, there is no existing reliable evidence that this regimen will affect chemical intolerance.

IMMUNOTHERAPY WITH CHEMICALS

Antibodies (both IgG and IgE) have been found in patients with specific chemical sensitivities, such as to trimellitic anhydride or toluene diisocyanate.[17] Recently such specific antibodies have also been found in formaldehyde-exposed subjects, though their clinical significance remains unclear at this point.[92,147] Clinical ecologists have proposed that broad chemical sensitivities are also mediated by the immune system and as such should be amenable to immunotherapy in the same way that dust allergy is. Randolph introduced the notion of the treatment of chemical sensitivities with ethanol injections or sublingual drops in 1964.[97] He proposed serial dilution skin testing to arrive at a "neutralizing dose" that could subsequently be used to abort acute reactions to a wide range of petrochemicals without close structural relationships to ethanol. This method has been further detailed and expanded in articles by Dickey[36] and Galapeaux[47] in a textbook on clinical ecology. With similar rationale, Randolph[95] suggested treatment with injectable phenol for treatment of broad chemical sensitivities. In an extension of this idea, McGovern[79] proposed the use of neutralizing doses of phenyl compounds naturally occurring in foods in an attempt to vitiate acute reactions to foods by chemically sensitive patients. Morris[86] has used the same technique for the treatment of a specific chemical sensitivity to formaldehyde. Although these authors have published extensive clinical anecdotes in presenting their theories, more rigorous data validating their claims are lacking. Further, the use of carcinogens such as those found in car exhaust or formaldehyde for intradermal testing and injection therapy is unacceptable. Finally, the rationale for using ethanol or phenol as antigens to treat broad chemical intolerances has not been satisfactorially explained. Therefore, at this point chemical immunotherapy cannot be generally recommended.

SUMMARY

The syndrome of multiple chemical sensitivities has many manifestations and undoubtedly many causes. Treatment must be individualized based on a thorough psychosocial and biological diagnostic evaluation. Careful listening, as is usually the case, not only results in a more complete history but also serves a critical therapeutic purpose in cementing a trusting, working partnership. Family dynamics, and larger social concerns, such as litigation, may figure importantly as obstacles to rehabilitation if they are ignored in treatment planning. In chronically disabled patients, the importance of psychosocial interventions is even greater but should not eclipse attention to relevant medical interventions. The most basic physiologic manipulation involves a program of environmental avoidance. Such a program should be applied with caution since it is not without risks of inadvertent exacerbation of medical and psychologic disabilities. Therefore, from a medical perspective, interventions should focus on improving chemical tolerance by the appropriate application of first aid, chronohygiene, nutrition, psychophysiology, and correction of microbiological disruptions. Thorough investigation for intercurrent disease and its appropriate management is paramount. Attempts to treat the entire problem by isolating attention to one area or based on a single theory are likely to fail.

REFERENCES

1. Abrahamson PR: Sarah: A Sexual Biography. Albany, NY, State University of New York Press, 1984.
2. Adkinson NF: Environmental influences on the immune system and allergic reactions. Environ Hlth Perspectives 20:97, 1977.
3. American Academy of Allergy: Position statements: Controversial techniques. J Allergy 67:333, 1981.
4. American Society of Heating, Refrigerating and Air-Conditioning Engineers, Inc: ASHRAE Transactions, 1985. 91: Part 1B, pp 611–622.
5. Andersen P: The occurrence of antibodies against Candida albicans in sera from normal subjects. Danish Med Bull 15:277, 1968.
6. Associated Press: Tainted water a Bay State woe. New Haven Register. March 31, 1986, p 7.
7. Baker SM, Galland L: Evaluating and treating the environmentally sensitive "complex patient." North American Nutrition & Preventive Medicine Association. Inc., San Diego, California, presented January 17–18, 1987.
8. Balint M: The drug "doctor." In Scott WR, Volkart EH (eds): Medical Care—Readings in the Sociology of Medical Institutions. New York, John Wiley and Sons, Inc., 1966, pp 281–291.
9. Balla JI, Moriatis S: Knights in armour: A follow-up study of injuries and legal settlement. Med J Aust Aug. 22, 1970.

10. Bardana EJ: Formaldehyde: Hypersensitivity and irritant reactions at work and in the home. Immunology & Allergy Practice 2:60, 1980.
11. Barnes JM: Assessing hazards from prolonged and repeated low doses of toxic substances. Br Med Bull 31:196, 1975.
12. Bell IR: Clinical Ecology. Bolinas, California, Common Knowledge Press, 1982.
13. Benson H, Klipper MZ: The Relaxation Response. New York, Avon Books, 1975.
14. Bernade MA, Mayerson EW: Patient-physician negotiation. JAMA 239:1413, 1978.
15. Bokina AI, Eksler ND, Semenenko AD, et al: Investigation of the mechanism of action of atmospheric pollutants on the central nervous system and comparative evaluation of methods of study. Environ Health Perspectives 13:37, 1976.
16. Brodsky CM: 'Allergic to everything': a medical subculture. Psychosomatics 24:731, 1983.
17. Brooks SM: Bronchial asthma of occupational origin. *In* Rom WN (ed): Environmental and Occupational Medicine. Boston, Little, Brown and Company, 1983, pp 233–257.
18. Brown EA, Colombo NJ: The asthmogenic effect of odors, smells and fumes. Ann Allergy 12:14, 1954.
19. Brown HS, Bishop DR, Rowan CA: The role of skin absorption as a route of exposure for volatile organic compounds (VOCs) in drinking water. Am J Public Health 74:479, 1984.
20. Burgeson B: Woman in constant battle with environment. Fairpress 8: June 20, 1979, p A22.
21. Butcher BT, O'Neill CE, Reed MA, et al: Development and loss of toluene diisocyanate reactivity: immunological, pharmacologic, and provocative challenge studies. J Allergy Clin Immunol 70:231, 1982.
22. Calabrese EJ: Nutrition and Environmental Health: The Influence of Nutritional Status on Pollutant Toxicity and Carcinogenicity, Volume I: The Vitamins. New York, John Wiley & Sons, Inc., 1980.
23. Calabrese EJ: Nutrition and Environmental Health: The Influence of Nutritional Status on Pollutant Toxicity and Carcinogenicity, Volume II: Minerals and Macronutrients. New York, John Wiley & Sons, 1981.
24. Carlson E: Synergistic effect of Candida albicans and Staphylococcus aureus on mouse mortality. Infect Immun 38:921, 1982.
25. Chow CK: Nutritional influences on cellular antioxidant defense systems: Am J Clin Nutr 32:1066, 1979.
26. Collier R: Building a house for the chemically intolerant individuals. *In* Dickey LD (ed): Clinical Ecology. Springfield, Illinois, Charles C Thomas, 1976, pp 515–523.
27. Colligan MJ: Shiftwork: health and performance effects. *In* Rom WN (ed): Environmental and Occupational Medicine. Boston, Little, Brown and Company, 1983, pp 751–755.
28. Condie LW: Toxicological problems associated with chlorine dioxide. Journal of the American Water Works Association: June 1986, pp 73–78.
29. Cornish HH, Adefuin J: Ethanol potentiation of halogenated aliphatic solvent toxicity. AM J Ind Hyg 27:57, 1966.
30. Cross CE, Halliwell B, Allen A: Antioxidant protection: a function of tracheobronchial and gastrointestinal mucus. Lancet 1:1328, 1984.
31. Dadd DL: Non-toxic & Natural. Los Angeles, Jeremy P Tarcher, Inc., 1984.
32. Dadd DL: Special report: Air filters. Nontoxic & Natural Newsletter, 1985.
33. Davis M. Eshelman ER, McKay MS: The Relaxation & Stress Reduction Workbook, 2nd ed. Oakland, California, New Harbringer Publications, 1982.
34. De Nevers N: Community air pollution. *In* Rom WN (ed): Environmental and Occupational Medicine. Boston, Little, Brown and Company, 1983, pp 797–809.
35. Department of Health, Education and Welfare, Food and Drug Administration: Proposed rule making: bottled water, proposed quality standard. Federal Register, January 8, 1973, p 1019.
36. Dickey LD: Sublingual antigen testing and therapy for inhalants, foods, and petrochemicals. *In* Dickey LD (ed): Clinical Ecology. Springfield, Illinois, Charles C Thomas, 1976, pp 544–553.
37. Dillard CJ, Litov, RE, Savin WM, et al: Effects of exercise, vitamin E, and ozone on pulmonary function and lipid peroxidation. J Appl Physiol 45:927, 1978.
38. Doull J: Factors influencing toxicology. *In* Doull J, Klaassen, CD, Amdur, MO (eds): Casarett and Doull's Toxicology—The Basic Science of Poisons, 2nd ed. New York, Macmillan Publishing Co., Inc., 1980, pp 70–83.
39. Ehret CF: New Approaches to chronohygiene for the shift worker in the nuclear power industry. *In* Reinberg A, Vieus N, Andlauer P (eds): Night and Shift Work: Biological and Social Aspects. Advances in the Biosciences, Volume 30. Oxford, Pergamon Press, 1981, pp 263–270.

40. Empey DW, Laitnen LA, Jacobs L, et al: Mechanisms of bronchial hyper-reactivity in normal subjects after upper respiratory tract infections. Am Rev Respir Dis 113:131, 1976.
41. Engle GL: The need for a new medical model: a challenge for biomedicine. Science 196:129, 1977.
42. Everything Natural, Inverness CA 94937.
43. Federal Response to Health Risks of Formaldehyde in Home Insulation, Mobile homes, and Other Consumer Products—hearings before a Subcommittee of the Committee on Government Operations, House of Representatives, Ninety-seventh Congress, Second Session. May 18 and 19, 1982. US Government Printing Office, Washington, 1982. pp 171–179.
44. Fine LJ: Occupational heart disease. In Rom WN (ed): Environmental and Occupational Medicine. Boston, Little, Brown and Company, 1983, p 361.
45. Friedman RD: Sensitive Populations and Environmental Standards. Washington, DC, The Conservation Foundation, 1981.
46. Friedson E: Client control and medical practice. In Jaco EG (ed): Patients, Physicians and Illness, New York, The Free Press, 1972, pp 211–214.
47. Galapeaux EA: Chemical testing and therapy. In Dickey LD (ed): Clinical Ecology. Springfield, Illinois, Charles C Thomas, 1976, pp 402–407.
48. Galland L: Nutrition and candida albicans. In Bland J (ed): The year in Nutritional Medicine—1986. New Canaan, Connecticut, Keats Publishing Inc. (in press).
49. Golos N, Golbitz FG: If This is Tuesday, It Must be Chicken, or How to Rotate Your Food for Better Health. Dallas, Human Ecology Research Foundation of Southwest, 1981.
50. Gyntelberg F, Vesterhauge S, Fog P, et al: Acquired intolerance to organic solvents and results of vestibular testing. Am J Indust Med 9:363, 1986.
51. Hart RA: Modification of an existing home. In Dickey LD (ed): Clinical Ecology. Springfield, Illinois, Charles C Thomas, 1976, pp 524–534.
52. Hazardous flouride levels in Napa Valley mineral waters. Nontoxic & Natural News 2:1, January 1986.
53. Hobbs CH, McClellan RO: Radiation and radioactive materials. In Doull J, Klaassen CD, Amdur MO (eds): Cassarett and Doull's Toxicology—The Basic Science of Poisons, 2nd ed. New York, Macmillan Publishing Co., Inc. 1980, p 510.
54. Hochman G: Allergic to everything. Health 56, March 1986.
55. Hoffman RE, et al: Health effects of long term exposure to 2,3,7,8-tetrachlorodibenzo-pdioxin. JAMA 255:2031, 1986.
56. Iwata K: A review of the literature on drunken symptoms due to yeasts in the gastrointestinal tract. In Iwata K (ed): Yeasts and Yeast-like Microorganisms in Medical Science. Tokyo, University of Tokyo Press, 1972, pp 259–268.
57. Karnovsky ML: Progress in sleep. N Engl J Med 315:1026, 1986.
58. Kasl SV: The health belief model and behavior related to chronic illness. Hlth Educ Monog 2:433, 1974.
59. Kasl SV, Cobb S: Health behavior, illness behavior and sickrole behavior. Arch Environ Hlth 12:246–265, 531, 541, 1966.
60. Keough, C: Water fit to drink. Emmaus, PA, Rodale Press, 1980.
61. King DS: Can allergic exposure provoke psychological symptoms? A double-blind test. Biol Psychiatry 16:333, 1981.
62. King J: Is your water safe to drink? Medical Self-Care 31:44, November/December 1985.
63. Klaassen CD: Absorption, distribution, and excretion of toxicants. In Doull J, Klaassen CD, Amdur MO (eds): Cassarett and Doull's Toxicology. New York, Macmillan Publishing Co., Inc., 1980, pp 28–55.
64. Komisaruk BR, Beyer C: Responses of diencephalic neurons to olfactory bulb stimulation, odor, and arousal. Brain Res 36:153, 1972.
65. Kunkel G, Rudolph R, Mulkelmann R: Indoor air and allergic diseases. Schriftenr Ver Wasser Boden Lufthys 53:75, 1982 (German with English abstract).
66. Kuvaeva IB, Orlova NU, Veselova OL, et al: Microecology of the gastrointestinal tract and the immunological status under food allergy. Nahrung 28:689, 1984.
67. Lafavore M: Clean air indoors. Rodale's New Shelter May/June:20, 1982.
68. Levin LS, Katz AH, Holst E: Self-care—Lay Initiatives in Health, New York, Prodist, 1976.
69. Levine RJ, Romm FJ, Sexton DJ, et al: Outbreak of psychosomatic illness at a rural elementary school. Lancet ii:1150, 1974.
70. Levine SA, Kidd PM: Antioxidant Adaptation—Its Role in Free Radical Pathology. San Leandro, CA, Biocurrents Division Allergy Research Group, 1985.

71. Likoff R, Nockels C, et al: Vitamin E and aspirin depress prostaglandin in protection of chickens against Escherichia coli infection. Am J Clin Nutr 34:245, 1981.
72. Liska B, Stadelman W: Accelerated removal of pesticides from domestic animals. Residue Rev 29:51, 1969.
73. Locke SE: Psychological and Behavioral Treatments for Disorders Associated with the Immune System, an Annotated Bibliography. New York, Institute for the Advancement of Health, 1986.
74. Locke SE, Hornig-Rohan M: Mind and Immunity: Behavioral Immunology, an Annotated Bibliography 1976–1982. New York, Institute for the Advancement of Health, 1983.
75. Luce GG: Biological Rhythms in Human & Animal Physiology. New York, Dover Publications, Inc., 1971.
76. Luster MI, Faith RE: Assessment of immunologic alteration caused by halogenated aromatic hydrocarbons. Ann NY Acad Sci 320: 1979.
77. Mathur S, Melchers JT, Ades EW, et al: Anti-ovarian and anti-lymphocyte antibodies in patients with chronic vaginal candidiasis. J Reprod Immunol 2:247, 1980.
78. Mauch H: Diagnostic value of monitoring kinetics of antibody responses in candidiasis by a solid-phase radioimmunoassay. Am J Clin Path 79:200, 1983.
79. McGovern JJ, Gardner RW, Brenneman LD, et al: Role of naturally occurring haptens in allergy. Ann Allergy 47:123, 1981.
80. McLellan RK: Health hazards of office work. Toxic Substances Journal 5:162, 1984.
81. McLellan RK: Enabling the disabled. Paper presented at Yeast-Human Interaction, San Francisco, March 30, 1985.
82. Metz SA: Anti-inflammatory agents as inhibitors of prostaglandin synthesis in man. Med Clin N Am 65:713, 1981.
83. Miller MH: Accident Neurosis. Br Med J: 919–925, 992–998, 1961.
84. Milner PM: Physiological Psychology. New York, Holt, Rinehart and Winston, Inc., 1970, pp 137–146.
85. Miner HR: Total environmental control for the ecologically ill and other patients with respiratory problems. In Dickey LD (ed): Clinical Ecology. Springfield, Illinois, Charles C Thomas, 1976, pp 535–543.
86. Morris DL: Recognition and treatment of formaldehyde sensitivity. Clinical Ecology 1:27, 1982.
87. Moses M: Pesticides. In Rom WN: Environmental and Occupational Medicine. Boston, Little, Brown and Company, 1983, pp 547–571.
88. Moses M, Lilis R, Crow KD, et al: Health status of workers with past exposure to 2,3,7,8-tetrachlorodibenzo-p-dioxin in the manufacture of 2,4,5-trichlorophenoxyacetic acid: comparison of findings with and without chloracne. Am J Ind Med 5:161, 1984.
89. Muranaka M, Suzuki S, Koizumi K, et al: Adjuvant activity of diesel-exhaust particulates for the production of IgE antibody in mice. J Allergy Clin Immunol 77:616, 1986.
90. Nisson N: Health and humidity. Rodale's New Shelter, April 1986, pp 12–15.
91. Parsons T: The Social System. New York, The Free Press, 1951.
92. Patterson R, Pateras V, Grammer LC, Harris KE: Human antibodies against formaldehyde-human serum albumin conjugates or human serum albumin in individuals exposed to formaldehyde. Int Arch Allergy Appl Immun 79:53, 1986.
93. Philpott WH: Methods of relief of acute and chronic symptoms of deficiency-allergy-addiction maladaptive reaction to foods and chemicals. In Dickey LD (ed): Clinical Ecology. Springfield, Illinois, 1976, pp 496–509.
94. Porter WP, Hinsdill R, Fairbrother A, et al: Toxicant-disease-environment interaction associated with suppression of immune system, growth and reproduction. Science 224:1014, 1984.
95. Randolph TG: Human Ecology and Susceptibility to the Chemical Environment. Springfield, Illinois, Charles C Thomas 1978.
96. Randolph TG: The enzymatic, acid, hypoxia, endocrine concept of allergic inflammation. In Dickey LD (ed): Clinical Ecology. Springfield, Illinois, Charles C Thomas, 1976, pp 577–596.
97. Randolph TH, Moss RW: An Alternative Approach to Allergies. New York, Lippincott & Crowell, Publishers, 1980.
98. Rea WJ: Environmentally triggered cardiac disease. Ann Allergy 40:243, 1978.
99. Rea WJ: Environmentally triggered small vessel vasculitis. Ann Allergy 38:245, 1977.
100. Rea WJ: Environmentally triggered thrombophlebitis. Ann Allergy 37:101, 1976.
101. Rea WJ, Bell IR, Suits CW, Smiley RE: Food and chemical susceptibility after environmental chemical overexposure: case histories. Ann Allergy 41:101, 1978.
102. Rea WJ, Butler JR, Johnson AR, et al: Pesticides and brain function changes in a controlled environment. Clinical Ecology 11:145, 1984.

103. Regtop H: Nutrition, leukotrienes and inflammatory disorders. *In* Bland J (ed): 1984–1985 Yearbook of Nutritional Medicine. New Canaan, Connecticut, Keats Publishing, Inc. 1985, pp 55–70.

104. Reinberg A: The hours of changing responsiveness or susceptibility. Perspect Bio Med 11:111–128, 1967.

105. Reinberg A, Sidi E, Ghata J: Circadian reactivity rhythms of human skin to histamine or allergen and the adrenal cycle. J Allergy 36:273–283, 1965.

106. Reinberg A, Vieux N, Andlauer P (eds): Night and Shift Work: Biological and Social Aspects. Advances in the Biosciences, Volume 30, Oxford, Pergamon Press, 1981.

107. Rinkel HJ, Randolph TG, Zeller M: Food Allergy. Norwalk, Connecticut, NE Foundation for Allergic and Environmental Diseases, 1976.

108. Rodale's Allergy Relief, 33 E. Minor St, Emmaus, PA 18049.

109. Rogers SA: When your home makes you sick - a physician's view of environmental illness. Bestways, February 1985, pp 8, 11.

110. Rogers TJ, Balish E: Immunity to Candida albicans. Microbiol Rev 44:660, 1980.

111. Rosenman KD: Cardiovascular disorders. *In* Levy BS, Wegman DH (eds): Occupational Health. Boston, Little, Brown and Company, 1983, pp 331–340.

112. Rozman K, Rozman T, Greim H: Enhanced fecal elimination of stored hexachlorobenzene from rats and rhesus monkeys by hexadecane or mineral oil. Toxicol 22:33, 1981.

113. Rudin DO: Omega-3 essential fatty acids in medicine. *In* Bland J (ed): 1984–1985 Yearbook of Nutritional Medicine. New Canaan, Connecticut, Keats Publishing, Inc. 1985, pp 37–54.

114. Schnare DW, Ben M, Shields MG: Body burden reductions of PCB's, PBB's and chlorinated pesticides in human subjects: Ambio 13(5–6):378–380, 1984.

115. Schnare DW, Denk G, Shields M, Brunton S: Evaluation of a detoxification regimen for fat stored xenobiotics. Med Hypoth 9:265, 1982.

116. Schottenfeld RS, Cullen MR: Recognition of occupation-induced post-traumatic stress disorders. J Occup Med 28:365, 1986.

117. Schwartz G, Beatty J (eds): Biofeedback Theory and Research. New York, Academic Press, 1977.

118. Schwartz GE: personal communication, 1986.

119. Seelig MS: Mechanisms by which antibiotics increase the incidence and severity of candidiasis and alter the immunological defenses. Bacteriological Rev 30:442, 1966.

120. Shim C, Williams MH: Effects of odors in asthma. Am J Med 80:18, 1986.

121. Siniscalchi A, Acting Director of Toxic Hazards, Connecticut State Department of Health Services. Personal communication, 1985.

122. Smilkstein G: The family APGAR: a proposal for a family function test and its use by physicians. J Fam Pract 6:1231, 1978.

123. Sohnle PG, Collins-Lech C, Huhta KE: Class-specific antibodies in young and aged humans against organism-producing superficial fungal infections. Brit J Derm 108:69, 1983.

124. Spiro HM: Clinical Gastroenterology, 2nd ed. New York, Macmillan Publishing Co., Inc., 1977, p 498.

125. Sprince H, Parker CM, Smith GG: Comparison of protection by l-ascorbic acid, l-cysteine, and adrenergic-blocking agents against acetaldehyde, acrolein, and formaldehyde toxicity: implications in smoking. Agents Actions 9:407–414, 1979.

126. Steinbergs CZ: Removal of by-products of chlorine and chlorine dioxide at a hemodialysis center. Journal of the American Water Works Association:June 1986, pp 94–98.

127. Stellman J, Henifin MS: Office Work Can Be Dangerous to Your Health. Nw York, Pantheon Books, 1983.

128. Stellman JM, Klitzman S, Gordon GC, Snow BR: Air quality and ergonomics in the office: Survey results and methodologic issues. Am Ind Hyg Assoc J 46:286–293, 1985.

129. Stevenson DD: Asthma. *In* Lockey RF (ed): Allergy & Clinical Immunology. Garden City, New York, Medical Examination Publishing Co., Inc., 1979, pp 712–761.

130. Stoeckle JD, Zola IK, Davidson GE: On going to see the doctor: the contributions of the patient to the decision to seek medical aid. J Chron Dis 16:975, 1963.

131. Street J: Methods of removal of pesticide residues. Can Med Ass J 100:16, 1969.

132. Sulfites in drugs and foods. Medical Letter 28:74, 1986.

133. Supramaniam G, Warner JO: Artificial food additive intolerance in patients with angio-edema and urticaria. Lancet ii:906, 1986.

134. Sweet LC: Toluene diisocyanate asthma. Univ. Mich Med J 34:27, 1968.

135. Szasz TS, Hollender MH: A contribution to the philosophy of medicine—the basic models of the doctor-patient relationship. Arch Intern Med 97:585, 1956.
136. Terr AI: Environmental illness—a clinical review of 50 cases. Arch Intern Med 146:145, 1986.
137. Torrey EF: The Mind Game. New York, Bantam Books, 1973.
138. Trimble MR: Post-Traumatic Neurosis—From Railway Spine to the Whiplash. New York, John Wiley & Sons, 1981.
139. Truss CO: Metabolic abnormalities in patients with chronic candiasis. J Orthomol Psychiatry 13:66, 1984.
140. Truss CO: Restoration of immunologic competence to Candida albicans. J Orthomol Psychiatry 9:287, 1980.
141. Truss CO: The role of Candida albicans in human illness. J Orthomol Psychiatry 10:228, 1981.
142. Truss CO: Tissue injury induced by Candida albicans: Mental and neurologic manifestations. J Orthomol Psychiatry 7:17, 1978.
143. Valnet J: The Practice of Aromatherapy. New York, Inner Traditions, 1982.
144. Water filters. Consumer Reports. February 1983, p 68.
145. Weed L: The problem oriented medical record as a basic tool in medical education and clinical research. Ann Clin R 3:131, 1971.
146. White KL, et al: The ecology of medical care. N Engl J Med 265:885, 1961.
147. Wojdani A, Thrasher JD, Heuser G, Cheung GP: Humoral and cellular immunity and IgG antibodies in humans chronically exposed to low concentrations of formaldehyde. Arch Env Hlth (in press).
148. Wood RW: Stimulus properties of inhaled substances. Environ Health Perspect 26:69, 1978.
149. Yagi K (ed): Lipid Peroxides in Biology and Medicine. New York, Academic Press, 1982.
150. Yudkin S: Six children with coughs—the second diagnosis. Lancet 561, 1961.
151. Zola IK: Culture and symptoms. Am Soc Rev 31:615, 1966.
152. Zola IK: Studying the decision to se a doctor. Adv Psychosom Med 8:216, 1972.
153. Zola IK: Pathways to the doctor—from person to patient. Soc Sci Med 7:677, 1973.

STEPHEN M. HESSL, MD, MPH

MANAGEMENT OF PATIENTS WITH MULTIPLE CHEMICAL SENSITIVITIES AT OCCUPATIONAL HEALTH CLINICS

Treatment of patients with multiple chemical sensitivities (MCS) often receives less attention by clinicians in occupational health clinics than diagnostic evaluation. Whether this is due to inadequate knowledge of how to treat such patients or to some frustration because these patients are "difficult," the lack of treatment as a priority is an error that prolongs the patient's symptoms and impairments. In fact, efforts to treat these patients should begin on the first visit to the occupational health clinic, before evaluation is complete, definitive diagnosis made, or the etiology of the problem is known. Furthermore, the treatment should be directed to the chronic aspects of the problem, and, in many instances, should involve other disciplines in addition to the occupational medicine physician, such as social services, occupational therapy, physical therapy, psychological counseling and vocational rehabilitation.

By the time the patient with MCS first visits the occupational health clinic, he or she is likely to have had multiple examinations at other health facilities with variable results. In spire of numerous previous attempts by the patient to obtain care for the problem, and often expensive and protracted workups, important diagnostic information may not have been ascertained. Therefore, the treatment of patients with MCS must always begin with a thorough review of the history, physical examination and diagnostic tests already performed. The staff of the occupational health clinic must incorporate into their interpretation of the problem an understanding that these patients have often already had multiple diagnoses (both accurate and inaccurate), multiple diagnostic tests (both necessary and unnecessary), and that the patients' lives may be in considerable turmoil (both cause and effect of the problem). Furthermore, the patient may already have alienated family, friends, personal physician, and employer, and had major changes in income, life style, and attitudes toward work.

The patients who have had the onset of their problems after an acute event, such as a spill, fire or other accidental overexposure in the workplace, frequently appear in the occupational health clinic days, weeks, and even months later. Other patients with MCS do not describe an acute episode such as an accidental contamination of the workplace or introduction of a new chemical into the workplace, nor does evidence of such an acute event commonly come to light even after a diligent attempt by the clinic staff to uncover a possible overexposure. In either

Division of Occupational Medicine, Cook County Hospital, Chicago, Illinois

Reprint requests to Stephen M. Hessl, MD, MPH, Division of Occupational Medicine, Cook County Hospital, Chicago, IL 60612 circumstance efforts are invariably directed to the chronic sequelae, focusing on the patient's current complaints and impairment. The discussion of the emergency management of acute toxic exposures which may subsequently lead to MCS is left to other excellent sources.[9,11,20,23]

The treatment of patients with MCS often requires techniques and services not routinely offered by primary care physicians. A multidisciplinary approach utilizing the skills of the social worker, psychologist, physical therapist, occupational therapist, vocational rehabilitation counselor, and others is often useful and necessary to develop and implement a successful treatment plan. Since many of these support staff may not be aware of the special problems and difficulties in managing patients with MCS, it is important to provide regular "in service" educational sessions on the subject for these support staff. Frequent group discussions about these patients should be convened in order to assure that a cohesive treatment plan is offered to the patient, which provides support to the patient in dealing with family, employer, co-workers, attorneys, insurance carriers and others, and provides specific therapies to modify the patient's symptoms and reactions to perceived injuries or exposures.

As mentioned above, the efforts to manage the myriad of problems that encircle the patient with MCS must begin on the first visit to the occupational health clinic. For example, reinforcement of positive, "well" behavior should begin on the first encounter with the patient. Although adequate history-taking requires attention to negative factors, such as the patient's symptoms and disability, attention should also be given to any positive factors such as success, however minimal, the patient may have had in coping with his/her problems. The occupational health clinic staff should obtain information from the patient about the circumstances that alleviate symptoms and about interests and activities that generate a sense of accomplishment or pleasure for the patient. To emphasize this, visits to the clinic should be scheduled frequently and regularly rather than in response to necessarily negative crisis situations. During subsequent visits, further attention should be given to the accomplishments by the patient or other positive experiences and "well" behaviors in addition to the necessary review of complaints, physical examinations and laboratory tests. If follow-up visits are on a "prn" basis, the patient will select times when increase in symptoms have occurred. That timing will encourage negative, "sick" behavior and inhibit efforts by the clinic staff to reinforce "well" behavior.

INDIVIDUAL TREATMENT METHODS

There is a wide variety of available therapies that can be attempted to alleviate symptoms and/or modify the negative behavior patterns of patients with MCS. Many of the techniques are borrowed from the management of problems that are similar to and overlap those of the patient with MCS. These problems include the post traumatic stress disorder,[1] chronic pain syndromes,[27] depression,[1] and somatoform disorders.[1] These interventions include both pharmacologic and psychologic methods, as listed in Table 1.

The fact that there are so many treatments available reflects the difficulty with management of patients with these conditions, the differing opinions regarding the etiology of the conditions, and the experience that no single modality is effective in all situations. If highly effective treatment were available which met the patient's needs and satisfied the physician's desires for consistent, objective improvement, such a wide variety of treatments would not be necessary. The fact that so many methods have been attempted is prima facie evidence that no single modality is effective in the majority of cases. The specific interventions should be chosen according to the nature of the patient's illness, the psychological status of the patient and the interest, training, skill, experience and success of the specialists available to provide the therapy. For example, hypnosis is not available to all occupational health clinics and is most effective in patients who are highly hypnotically suggestible.[6]

It is not practical or necessary to refer all patients with known or suspected multiple chemical sensitivities for therapies such as those listed in Table 1. Therefore, selection should occur in the occupational health clinic. The staff in the clinic must be familiar with the therapies and their indications. A set of criteria should be established for the clinic staff to use as an aid in selecting those patients who should be referred for further psychologic evaluation and possible treatment. Table 2 provides an example of indicators that are not exhaustive but may be useful to the clinic staff in making recommendations for further treatment.

If further psychological evaluation and treatment are recommended, accep-

TABLE 1. Interventions of Potential Value in Patients with Multiple Chemical Sensitivities

INTERVENTION	POPULATION TESTED
Pharmacologic	
Imipramine	Post-traumatic stress[4]
Lithium	Post-traumatic stress[14]
Psychologic	
Psychotherapy	Post-traumatic stress[15]
Relaxation training	Migraine headaches[12]
	Tension headaches[25]
	Chronic low back pain[26]
	Myofascial pain[8]
Biofeedback	Migraine headaches[2]
	Tension headaches[3]
	Chronic musculoskeletal pain[16]
	Temporomandibular joint pain[7]
	Chronic low back pain[10]
Operant treatment	Chronic low back pain[17]
	Diverse syndromes[21]
Hypnosis	Migraine headaches[6]
	Cancer pain[22]
	Diverse syndromes[18]
	Post-traumatic headache[5]

TABLE 2.   Criteria for Psychological Consultation and Referral of Patients with Multiple Chemical Sensitivities

I.	DEPRESSION—Appetite or sleep disturbances, psychomotor agitation or retardation, decreased energy, feelings of worthlessness or guilt, difficulty concentrating, suicidal ideation.
II.	ANXIETY AND POST TRAUMATIC STRESS—Reexperiencing of the trauma, decreased involvement with or response to the outside world, hyperalertness, avoidance of activities which recall the event.
III.	SOMATIZATION—Sickliness, pseudoneurologic, cardiopulmonary, gastrointestinal, psychosexual, and pain symptoms.
IV.	CONVERSION—Pseudoneurologic signs and symptoms (e.g., paralysis, dyskinesia, paresthesia, pseudoseizures).
V.	HYPOCHONDRIASIS—Unrealistic interpretation of physical signs or sensations as abnormal.
VI.	Other indications of difficulty coping with the illness or exposure(s).

tance by the patient is frequently a problem for the occupational health clinic. The patient with MCS often is convinced of an organic basis for the symptoms and denies the psychological factors that frequently play a role in the illness. Since many of the treatments imply a psychological component to the illness and are usually conducted by psychologists or psychiatrists, the patient may be reluctant to participate for fear of being labeled as psychologically unfit in some way. This is a delicate matter that requires considerable skill to overcome on the part of the clinic staff. One method that frequently is useful in overcoming this obstacle takes advantage of the fact that these patients frequently will accept further diagnostic testing. Neurobehavioral testing often provides an accepted avenue to introduce the concept that there may be a psychological component to the illness. These tests may demonstrate objective abnormalities in performance which are based on specific nervous system effects due to exposure to metals, solvents, and other hazards to which the patient may have been exposed.[13] In addition, the testing may demonstrate abnormalities more likely to be due to psychological factors such as anxiety or depression. This information is not only useful from a diagnostic standpoint, but will also assist in selecting the most appropriate treatment and in providing data that may help to objectively demonstrate to the patient that there is a psychological component to the illness. As a result of the encounter with the staff administering the neurobehavioral tests, the patient may begin to develop some acceptance of psychological factors and some confidence in the professionals involved. As a result, the patient may be more receptive to subsequent therapy using methods such as those listed in Table 1.

Since the interventions listed in Table 1 have been used and tested in various populations, which may overlap with but are not synonymous with the patients with MCS, strong consideration should be given to developing clinical trials to demonstrate the effectiveness of the techniques in these patients. Future studies are essential to determine the most effective treatments and to more clearly define the associated syndromes of patients with MCS.

SOCIAL CONTEXT

In addition to the pharmacologic and psychologic interventions listed in Table 1, appropriate management of the patient with multiple chemical sensitivities requires a full understanding of the patient's interactions with his social environment. It must be emphasized that the entire clinic staff should have as complete an understanding of the social interactions of the patient as possible. The staff must have skill in providing support in the patient's relationships with family, employer, coworkers, legal advocates, other health providers and insurance carriers. Because the symptoms are nonspecific, the physical examination unremarkable, and the laboratory tests are inconclusive, the diagnosis may be unclear and the specific etiology of the condition may be undefined. As a result, the patient's complaints are often viewed with skepticism and received with hostility by those with whom he or she interacts, including other health professionals. Lack of sympathy and negative reactions by others often complicate the patient's life and the clinic's effort to manage the patient by alienating the patient, aggravating any associated anxiety or depression, and prolonging the period of disability. The clinic staff must therefore be alert to these problems and provide appropriate support to minimize these problems.

The patient's interaction with the employer is often especially troublesome. The clinic staff must take great care to communicate appropriately with the employer and accurately advise the patient regarding the work-relatedness of the condition and the recommended work restrictions. In several respects the patient's outcome may depend on factors related to the workplace. Most importantly, exposures at work may be causal or contributing factors to the development of the illness.

If the patient's illness was caused by chemical exposures in the workplace, for example organic solvents, it is expected that ongoing exposures, even to low levels, may continue to cause symptoms and prolong the illness.[28] In such circumstances the patient should be removed from all exposure to the putative agents until the problems are resolved. In less severe cases, it may be prudent to recommend appropriate personal protective devices such as gloves and respirators. But the physician, patient and employer must keep in mind that such equipment does not provide complete protection.

Even when an organic basis for the patient's complaints is not identified, removal from exposure to the alleged offending chemicals may be advisable. For example, post-traumatic stress disorder may result from a real or imagined toxic exposure in the workplace. Even though an accident or spill at the workplace may have been the precipitating event, the patient with post-traumatic stress disorder may continue to suffer from symptoms for many months afterwards.[24] The chronic nature of the disorder, as well as resistance by the employer in accepting the claims of the patient, often leads to litigation in order for the patient to receive compensation for lost earnings and medical expenses. Negative relations with the employer, insurance carriers and company attorneys often ensue, which may aggravate associated anxiety and depression. Frequently, such patients are unjustly labeled as malingerers or accident neurotics, terms that have no diagnostic validity, are pejorative and further alienate the patient.[19]

Often, the patient already has made a decision not to work by the time of the initial visit to the occupational health clinic. This may have been on the basis of recommendations of physicians who previously evaluated the patient or an independent decision by the patient. The basis for the decision and previous communications with the employer must be reviewed to obtain a clear understanding of the employment status of the patient.

If the patient stops working without adequate justification, without a clear statement of the necessity for removal from exposure, without a description of the likely consequences of re-exposure and without a definition of the objectives, the employer is more likely to be unsympathetic. This can result in efforts by the employer to terminate the patient's employment or benefits. Such lack of clarity can also complicate any future efforts for the patient to receive compensation. Consequently, the patient may lose his job and suffer further loss of wages and self-esteem. The patient may remain at home with little to occupy his/her time except for concern about his/her health and future. Family and friends may become alienated.

Such a scenario is common for the patient with MCS and often aggravates associated anxiety and depression. The occupational health clinic must therefore take steps to avoid troublesome relations with the employer. Communications with the employer must be extremely clear, specific and in writing. If the patient came to the clinic on his own or was referred by someone other than his employer, appropriate consent must be given by the patient to communicate with the employer. Non-occupational illnesses should not be revealed to the employer. If a work-related disease is diagnosed, it should be clearly stated. Any work restrictions that may be advisable, regardless of etiology, should be indicated, as well as the duration of the recommendations. The anticipated consequences of continued exposure or noncompliance with the recommendations should be specified.

Examples of good and bad communications are shown in Figures 1 and 2. These letters demonstrate several important points that must be kept in mind when communicating with the patient's employer. While a "To whom it may concern" letter may be necessary if the patient does not know the name of the appropriate supervisor at work or if the patient has not given his consent to write directly to

FIGURE 1. "Bad" letter to employer.

OCCUPATIONAL MEDICINE CLINIC
YOUR CITY AND STATE
USA

To whom it may concern:

Mr. John Doe was evaluated in the Occupational Medicine Clinic on October 17. His diagnoses include high blood pressure, diabetes, and hypersensitivity to chemicals at work. His work exposures might have caused the problem, but it is not yet clear. He also has high blood pressure and diabetes which make it difficult to separate out which factor is causing his current symptoms.

Please move him to the Shipping Receiving area where he won't be exposed to the chemicals.

Sincerely,

FIGURE 2. "Good letter" to employer

OCCUPATIONAL MEDICINE CLINIC
YOUR CITY AND STATE
USA

Mr. John Smith
Supervisor of Furmulating Dept.
The Chemical Company

RE: John Doe

Dear Mr. Smith:

Mr. John Doe was evaluated in the Occupational Clinic on October 17, 1987 for a health problem which I believe is related to his chemical exposure at The Chemical Company. Diagnostic tests have been ordered for Mr. Doe which should help to clarify the nature and extent of his disease. In the meantime, I have advised Mr. Doe not to be exposed to any xylene, naptha, catalysts, or other volatile chemicals to which he had been exposed in the Formulating Department. Any further skin or respiratory exposure can be expected to aggravate his illness and prolong his convalescence.

Mr. Doe will be re-evaluated by me on November 14, 1987.

Sincerely,

cc: Mr. Doe

the employer, it is best to identify the manager who is responsible for the patient's work assignment and conditions. It is important to document communication to the employer to minimize confusion or misinterpretation about recommendations and to provide all parties a record for future medicolegal purposes. If the physician believes that the patient's symptoms or disease are related to work in some way, he or she should indicate that opinion to the employer even though the workup is not yet complete.

The physician should not include all of the doubts that he or she may have regarding the case. In Figure 1, the physician indicates that the patient's symptoms could be due to hypertension, diabetes, or the work experiences. Such a statement confuses the work-relatedness of the condition. If the work was an aggravating or contributing factor to the patient's illness, then a statement to that effect will suffice. The work does not have to be the sole cause of the patient's illness for the illness to be considered work-related and to justify appropriate work restrictions. Besides avoiding the confusion of the first letter, the second letter documents that the patient was advised of the work-relatedness of his/her illness and the recommended restrictions. The restrictions should be as specific as the circumstance will allow. If the physician has been able to ascertain the precise offending exposures in the workplace, these should be listed. Often, it is not possible to be so precise and words such as "solvents," "gases," "dusts," etc. must be substituted until the exact chemical names and forms of the compounds become available.

A statement about the permanency of the condition should also be considered. In the second letter, the patient was to be re-evaluated in one month, implying that the status might change at the time of follow-up. If the physician believes that the work-related condition or the work restrictions are permanent, he should indicate that to the employer.

The clinic is often requested to fill out insurance claim forms regarding the patient. Such forms should not be considered substitutes for direct communication with the employer. Furthermore, the forms often do not request the physician's opinion regarding specific work limitations. The physician should not limit his/her response to the yes/no questions on insurance forms and should provide a narrative whenever necessary to clarify the diagnosis, work restrictions, or prognosis.

PATIENT EDUCATION

Many of the educational efforts listed in Table 3 reinforce to the patient that he or she is not powerless to modify the factors that may have contributed to the illness. Education provides a potential means to promote "well" behavior and prevent further illness. It also provides tools for the patient to control his or her environment rather than encourage continued illness, disability and hopelessness.

Patients with MCS often have considerable anxiety about real or imagined health effects from chemical exposures at work and elsewhere. These patients frequently fear serious, adverse health outcomes such as cancer or severe debilitating disease as a consequence of their contact with potentially hazardous sub-

TABLE 3. Educational Goals for the Patient with Multiple Chemical Sensitivities

1. General Principles of Toxicology
    a. Routes of absorption and elimination of toxins
    b. Dose/response relationships.
    c. Acute versus chronic toxicity
    d. Hypersensitivity versus direct toxicity
2. Industrial Hygiene Measures
    a. Personal protective devices
    b. Engineering controls
    c. Environmental and biological monitoring
3. Host Factors
    a. Variations in susceptibility to disease
    b. Cigarettes, alcohol, diet and other "lifestyle" factors
4. Community and Other Resources
    a. OSHA
    b. EPA
    c. Lung Association
    d. Department of Public Health
    e. Unions
    f. Vocational Rehabilitation
    g. Workers Compensation

stances. They frequently avoid seemingly trivial exposures, claiming that these alleged contacts are harmful and cause uncomfortable symptoms. Sometimes the patient's complaints are bizarre and defy rational explanation or scientific inquiry.

In such a setting the occupational health clinic staff has the challenging task of determining the nature and physiologic consequences of the alleged exposure and of modifying the patient's response to the offending exposures. Since the patient may have already received different opinions regarding diagnosis, work-relatedness of the illness, degree of impairment and prognosis, he or she may be skeptical and unwilling to accept the clinic's analysis of the problem.

Doubts expressed by the clinic staff may be interpreted by the patient as trivializing the condition in some way, or not believing the patient is ill. Since the medical literature on MCS is incomplete, the physician frequently expresses doubt. The patient may even suspect that the physician is working in concert with the employer to the patient's detriment. Consequently, it is extremely important that the patient be given an opportunity to express these concerns and to be asked what his/her thoughts are in regard to the exposures and the anticipated outcomes. The clinic staff must reassure the patient and hopefully dispel irrational fears that may have developed.

Education does not necessarily lead to a change in behavior or attitudes, but the clinic staff must sedulously transmit their knowledge to the patient in a manner which will optimize the patient's understanding of the known versus implausible health effects expected as a consequence of their real versus imagined exposures. These educational efforts should embrace the subjects listed in Table 3 so that the patient may place his or her health problems into an objective context. For example, a patient may erroneously believe that a solvent with a relatively short half-life remains in the body for a long time and continues to cause damage. It may be a considerable relief for the patient to know that the substance was eliminated from the body long ago and should not be producing any further organ system damage long after the exposure ceased.

Other educational efforts include information about industrial hygiene measures available to reduce exposures. This may enable the patient to improve work practices and return to work with some confidence that exposures have been minimized. Similarly, information about routes of exposure as well as the importance of particle size, chemical composition, etc. in determining toxicity of a specific substance may enable the patient to make rational decisions about work status and prevent the patient from concluding that an exposure occurred when in fact little or no exposure was possible. Information about interactions of other exposures such as cigarettes, ethanol and diet may be important to reinforce "well" behavior by the patient.

SUMMARY

The difficult task of managing patients with MCS requires a multidisciplinary effort involving the occupational medicine physician, social worker, occupational therapist, physical therapist, psychologist, vocational rehabilitation specialist, industrial hygienist, and other involved professionals. Important objectives of management include complete review of the history and clinical findings, appropriate choice of diagnostic tests, search for additional exposure information, emphasis of "well" behavior, health education of the patient and prevention of further illness. Because of the chronic nature of MCS and the difficulty many patients have in coping with MCS, pharmacologic and psychologic interventions should be considered. Interaction of the clinic with the patients employer, insurance carrier, or attorney must be carefully planned and communicated only after receiving the patient's informed consent. Patient education should include general principles of toxicology, industrial hygiene measures to reduce hazardous exposures, factors which may aggravate the illness, and resources available to obtain further information and assistance.

REFERENCES

1. American Psychiatric Association: Diagnostic and Statistical Manual, 3rd ed. Washington, D.C., APA, 1980, pp 210–252.
2. Blanchard EB, et al: Temperature biofeedback in the treatment of migraine headaches. Arch Gen Psychiatry 35:581, 1978.
3. Budzynski TH, et al: EMG biofeedback and tension headache—A controlled outcome study. Psychosom Med 35:484, 1973.
4. Burstein A: Treatment of post-traumatic stress disorder with imipramine. Psychosomatics 24:681, 1984.
5. Cedercreutz C, et al: Self-regulation of pain, the use of alpha-feedback and hypnotic training for the control of chronic pain. Exp Neurol 24:195, 1976.
6. Friedman H, Taub HA: Brief psychological procedures in migraine treatment. Am J Clin Hypn 26:187, 1984.
7. Funch DP, Gale EN: Biofeedback and relaxation therapy for chronic temporomandibular joint pain—predicting successful outcomes. J Consult Clin Psychol 52:928, 1984.
8. Gessel AH, Alderman M: Management of myofascial pain dysfunction syndrome of the temporomandibular joint by tension control training. Psychosomatics 12:302, 1971.
9. Goldfrank LR, et al: Goldfrank's Toxicologic Emergencies, 3rd ed. Norwalk, Appleton-Century-Crofts, 1986, pp 1–929.
10. Gottlieb HG, et al: Low back pain comprehensive rehabilitation problem—A follow-up study. Arch Phys Med Rehabil 63:458, 1982.
11. Haddad LM, Winchester JF: Clinical Management of Poisoning and Drug Overdose. Philadelphia, WB Saunders, 1983, pp 1–1012.
12. Hay KM, Madders J: Migraine treated by relaxation therapy. J R Coll Gen Pract 21:664, 1971.
13. Johnson BL, Anger WK: Behavioral toxicology. In Rom WM: Environmental and Occupational Medicine. Boston, Little, Brown and Company, 1983, pp 329–350.
14. Kitchner I, Greenstein R: Low dose lithium carbonate in the treatment of post-traumatic stress disorder—Brief communication. Milit Med 150:378, 1985.
15. Kolb LC: Treatment of chronic post-traumatic stress disorders. Curr Psychiatr Ther 23:119, 1986.
16. Large RG, Lamb AM: Electromyographic (EMG) feedback in chronic musculoskeletal joint pain—A controlled trial. Pain 17:167, 1983.
17. Linton SJ, Gotestam KG: A controlled study of the effects of applied relaxation and applied relaxation plus operant procedures in the regulation of chronic pain. Br J Clin Psychol 23:291, 1984.
18. Melzack R, Perry C: Self-regulation of pain, the use of alpha-feedback and hypnotic training for the control of chronic pain. Exp Neurol 46:452, 1975.
19. Mendelson G: "Compensation Neurosis": An invalid diagnosis. Med J Aust 142:561, 1985.
20. Proctor NH, Hughes JP: Chemical Hazards of the Workplace. Philadelphia, JB Lippincott, 1978, pp 1–533.

21. Roberts AH, Reinhardt L: The behavioral management of chronic pain—Long term follow-up with comparison groups. Pain 8:151, 1980.
22. Sacerdote P: Theory and practice of pain control in malignancy and other protracted or recurring painful illnesses. J Clin Exp Hypn 18:160, 1970.
23. Schwartz GR, et al: Principles and Practice of Emergency Medicine, 2nd ed. Philadelphia, WB Saunders, 1986, pp 1–1799.
24. Tarsh MJ, Royston C: A follow-up study of accident neurosis. Br J Psychiatry 146:18, 1985.
25. Tasto D, Hinkle JE: Muscle relaxation treatment for tension headaches. Behav Res Ther 11:347, 1973.
26. Turner JA: Comparison of group progressive-relaxation training and cognitive-behavioral group therapy for chronic low back pain. J Consult Clin Psychol 50:757, 1982.
27. Turner JA, Chapman CR: Psychological interventions for chronic pain—A clinical review I & II. Pain 12:1, 1982.
28. Winneke G: Acute behavioral effects of exposure to some organic solvents—Psycho-physiological aspects. ACTA Neurol Scand (suppl)92 66:117, 1982.

BETH M. LEWIS, MSW, ACSW, CISW

WORKERS WITH MULTIPLE CHEMICAL SENSITIVITIES: PSYCHOSOCIAL INTERVENTION

The patient with "multiple chemical sensitivities" presents a challenge for practitioners in the medical/occupational health setting. Given the nature of the illness, rooted as it is in the social/biological environment of the "20th century,"[10] interdisciplinary cooperation in practice is perhaps more essential to successful diagnosis, assessment and treatment with this group than for any other population currently seen as regularly in such settings. The value of this volume—an attempt to combine the knowledge bases and skills of the various professions sharing a common goal of helping such patients live satisfying and socially useful lives— is in reaching for a definition of the syndrome and exploring avenues of treatment for patients who, without such work, may continue to frustrate any single profession's intervention efforts.

Indeed, the frustration experienced by physicians who treat patients with multiple chemical sensitivities (MCS) is not a small part of the overall consideration given by social workers to the psychosocial aspects of this and other illnesses which "do not improve" with medical intervention.[8] The controversy raging within the medical-psychiatric-clinical ecology communities as to a definitive approach to diagnosis and treatment of MCS implies a set of psychosocial complications of the illness. Nevertheless, it is necessary, as a basis for further discussion of management techniques, to briefly summarize the diagnostic features of the syndrome, explicated at greater length in preceding chapters of this volume. For purposes of this article, and to save the reader any redundancy, the lengthy listing of exclusionary diagnoses/illnesses (both medical and psychiatric) will not be reviewed here and are accepted as given on the basis of colleagues' work in this area.

The syndrome of MCS typically involves a previous, documented environmental (including workplace) exposure, "insult," or illness. Symptoms related to such exposure persist and recur in relation to demonstrable, often extremely low-level, exposures that usually extend beyond those to which the patient originally reacted. The fact that the latter diagnostic feature is usually involved may often form the basis of concern for patients with MCS, causing a degree of restriction in life-style previously not experienced, thus resulting in a decision to seek medical help. As such restrictions—self-imposed or otherwise—are typically seen at the

From the Department of Social Work, Yale-New Haven Hospital, New Haven, Connecticut

Reprint requests to Beth M. Lewis, MSW, Department of Social Work, Yale-New Haven Hospital, New Haven, CT 06510.

time of presentation, the psychosocial aspect of the illness is invariably a component, rounding out the diagnosis of the syndrome.

Herein three elements emerge that involve the need for psychosocial assessment and intervention: (1) the occurrence of environmental* exposures, involving exploration of the "how, what and why" of such exposure; (2) the recurrence of symptoms on exposure to lower-level and usually ever-expanding environmental stimuli, involving perceived changes in the health of the individual; and (3) the restriction in life-style affecting patient as well as family members. The implications for psychosocial assessment and intervention in each of the above diagnostic areas will be discussed, utilizing case material as illustration of techniques used in practice.

THE SOCIAL REALITY OF THE WORKPLACE: A COMPONENT OF THE PSYCHOSOCIAL ASSESSMENT

A pioneer in industrial social work practice, who, earlier, began her career helping to lay the foundations of medical social work practice, has written:[9]

> The conditions under which people earn their living, or are prevented from doing so, determine their mindset toward life more than any individual differences.

While the underlying principle embodied in this statement stems from Reynolds' work with a different population at a different historical period from the present, it continues to provide invaluable direction for current-day thinking about practice with MCS patients and their families.

We live in a time of increasing technological advances, both in and outside of the workplace. In the face of such advances, workers everywhere live with the stress of continually having to make adjustments to new work processes. The by-products of these processes carry potentially greater promise for "stress" than the adjustments to the process itself, if for no other reason than that their effects on individual workers, by and large, have not been quantified, at least in a manner comprehensible to the lay person.[1] Along with making the adjustments must be added the stress of finding one's vocational skills outdated at an increasingly rapid rate, necessitating further education and/or training in order to compete in the workplace world.[6]

Finally, the economic scene, including the rising rate of unemployment for certain sectors of the workforce, a shift of resources from the public to the private sector, decreasing real wages, and erosion of protections and supports, both legislated and negotiated, combine to create a vise-like atmosphere. One might expect to find a certain portion of the workforce afflicted to varying degrees by the following set of reactions to the stressors mentioned previously: fear of the unknown; a sense of inadequacy, failure or lack of value placed on one's abilities; competitiveness

---

*We will focus on the workplace as the meaningful environmental agent in a discussion of the effect on the patient of workplace exposure.

with others for a share in the shrinking resources available to most; and anger and resentment over the increasing resources available to a few.[11] While the unorganized, blue-collar industrial worker may very well have potentially greater exposure to these stressors,[2,6] this set of circumstances forms the basis of the socioeconomic reality of most workers, regardless of the nature of their workplace or individual vocation. In the context of a discussion of the social reality of today's workforce, it does not come as a surprise that the population presenting with MCS—to the occupational health clinic, for example—comprises workers from a wide variety of workplaces, with accompanying wide variation in educational, skill and socioeconomic levels. Keeping in mind the effects of such social factors on individuals and families, the author will now examine the psychological effect on patients of workplace exposures leading to the development of MCS.

WORKPLACE EXPOSURE AND THE MCS PATIENT

Patients' reports of exposures leading to the development of MCS typically involve feelings of inability to maintain control over both the circumstances surrounding and/or leading up to the exposure, and the exposure itself, as well as his/her reactions to the exposure.

Case Example 1: Mr. S., a 57-year-old immigrant who spoke halting English, presented to clinic 2½ years following an acute exposure to toxic solvents, which had occurred during his work at a large manufacturing plant. He was married × 15 years to an American woman of similar ethnic descent. The couple was childless.

His symptoms included dizziness, nausea, light-headedness, skin irritation, burning sensations in his chest and throat, and hoarseness. He complained of having these symptoms, which had originally occurred acutely with relatively high levels of solvent exposure, whenever he was exposed to "chemicals" or irritant odors of any kind, including such things as cigarette smoke, cooking fumes, salt air, and (his wife's) perfume. He had come to the clinic at the suggestion of his regular doctor, who had given up on him because, according to the patient, "My symptoms should not 'be' any longer." The patient was seen by the social worker following a medical examination which revealed no organic basis for his symptoms. Mrs. S. took the role of interpreter for her husband, although in subsequent interviews with the patient alone, it became apparent that Mr. S. had adequate command of the language without an interpreter.

During the initial social work interview, exploration of the events leading to the exposure and the exposure itself revealed the following history: The patient had worked at this plant since the time of his immigration to the United States, some 17 years prior. His uncle had arranged for him to get the job, which was in a union shop with competitive pay rates, and which was populated with workers from his country of origin. He met his wife at the plant and married her shortly after immigrating. Generally, he had been satisfied with his job until shortly before his exposure, which happened during a period of massive lay-offs at the plant, when he had been assigned to work that was technically not in his designated job category. Unlike his former job, this work involved high-level exposure to solvents while cleaning out degreaser tanks, a job which he did without personal protection. He had made a half-hearted attempt to protest the assignment, although he never filed a grievance through the union, even though he knew this to be the correct avenue for changing his assignment. When nothing was done, either concerning the assignment or the problem of protection, he decided to continue working because he had been kept at his regular pay rate and because, "With no seniority I was afraid I would lose my job altogether" (if he protested). He also blamed his failure to take any action on his own behalf on the fact that he "couldn't speak the language." Prior to the acute exposure, he had been "feeling sick" from chronic lower-level (albeit still substantial) exposures, and had been worried about his ability to continue working. He related that at the time of his acute exposure he thought he "was going to die." Since the event, he had never been the same, although he did attempt to work, agreeing to "lay-off" periods (during which he received unemployment insurance benefits supplemented by workers' compensation payments) at various points when he would become too symptomatic to continue working. He had currently been on such a lay-off for three months and, for the first time in 2½ years, felt unable to return to the plant, expressing the feeling that his "disability" was great enough that he was considering early (disability) retirement. He was worried, however, as was his wife, that at his age he could not afford to live on whatever meager amount he might be entitled to from partial pension payments.

The social worker, noting that the acute exposure, as well as the periods of sickness leading up to it and his subsequent failure to improve, had clearly been a difficult and frightening experience, arranged for a follow-up interview to discuss further his feelings about what had happened. In this way, the social worker explained, they could better explore together a plan for the future that would make sense, given his age, health and financial situation. Mr. S. stated that he "wasn't sure what would come of talking" but was willing to give it a try. He requested to have his wife present, to which the social worker agreed, recognizing the level of his emotional dependency that had emerged in the course of the discussion about his problem.

This example is used to illustrate the emotional impact of workplace exposures on the individual with MCS. As an initial interview, it also illustrates the importance of "beginning where the client is."[4] Here an effort was made to offer psychological support with an illness that presents with a patient's expression of feelings of inability in handling his/her situation adequately. This support is offered, initially, by encouraging the patient to talk freely and to express feelings about the situation, particularly the "insult" (the medical phraseology lending itself to interpretation of the impact of workplace exposures on the MCS patient) that is felt to have precipitated the illness.

Much has been written on the importance of supportive intervention in "beginnings" with medically ill clients; social workers must recognize that the patients may be able to deal emotionally with a problem that is *related* to the illness, achieving some security that is sufficient to permit involvement with the illness process itself. Indeed, the ability of the patient to identify a related problem and to seek help with it is key in determining the appropriateness of social work intervention.[5] In supporting the MCS patient's capacity to express feelings about the workplace and gain mastery over these feelings, the worker helps the patient achieve the abililty to mobilize both inner and outer resources to accommodate to the real threat to security, which comes with a focus on the illness itself. Concerns projected onto the illness at this level might involve fears about one's future health and the possibility that these symptoms may signify the presence of a more serious disease process, the deeper sense of loss that comes with the loss of health, and feelings that the illness is a punishment for the patient's past or present wrong-doings. Helping patients receive entitlements, if they request such help and are unable to work, and other techniques of environmental modification may also fulfill the supportive roles of early intervention. Importantly, such work should not be carried out in isolation, as the patient needing this type of intervention is usually also in need of psychological support.

To summarize, early intervention with the MCS patient should be supportive in nature. The need to discuss and explore feelings associated with workplace exposure may be identified by the patient as the problem requiring immediate attention. The emphasis should not be on the development of *understanding* by the patient but rather on "reinforcing ego strengths through guidance, release of tension and through reassurance."[5] Group treatment may be suggested if the patient is felt to be appropriate for this modality.

RECURRENCE OF SYMPTOMS: A PROBLEM IN ADJUSTMENT

In a paraphrase of Margolis' work on the "Biodynamic View" in *Medicine*, Cockerill wrote:[3]

Our attention has been drawn to the fact that the symptoms that are usually regarded as the disease itself are actually only descriptive of the nature of a problem in adjustment and indicative of the particular way in which the individual is attempting to resolve it.

The "biodynamic view" in medicine, certainly an antecedent of the principles underlying the practice of medicine in the field of clinical ecology, is one that sees disease as an expression of the human organism's "lack of ease" in "resolving a conflict between itself and an inimical or hostile agent."[7] It is perhaps most useful as a model guiding our work with MCS patients. Reflecting further on the meaning of this view for the practice of medical social work, Cockerill goes on to write:[3]

We sometimes fail to recognize the real strength and capacity reflected in the symptomatic behavior of the individual which we may tend to view as evidence only of pathology or lack of adequacy.

Margolis echoes this sentiment in his writings: ". . . the wonder, literally, is not that occasionally the human organism fails to rebound, but that so often it does."[7]

The capacity of MCS patients to develop insight into the psychological un-derpinnings of their sensitivity to environmental exposures must be assessed care-fully in the process of offering psychological support and clarification (also known as "counseling"). Often, in the process of offering clarification aimed at helping the patient think more clearly, react more realistically, and plan more wisely for contact with environmental stimuli that can only be avoided at great personal sacrifice, the patient may be helped to develop insights into the nature of their problem. The group treatment modality, where patients are able to discuss their feelings about having MCS in an atmosphere of mutual aid and acceptance, may offer the opportunity for developing such insight.

> **Case Example 2:** In a group with three other patients with MCS, Ms. L., a 33-year-old unmarried patient, reacted sensitively to exhaust fumes from a car parked outside the building. The door leading to the parking lot had been left ajar by the group leader at the request of another patient who was sensitive to Ms. L.'s perfume. Her subsequent request to have the door closed stimulated group discussion about the meaning for each member of their individual "sensitivities," with the group reaching the concensus that their individual reactions were not dissimilar to individual levels of tolerance for certain types of people and their particular habits.[14]

The judgement of the worker as to the ability of patients with MCS to develop such insight would also figure into the overall differential diagnostic assessment, involving the possible need for evaluation of psychiatric illness. Psychiatric consultation/evaluation and/or treatment would not necessarily preclude on-going social casework services. Psychiatric therapeutic intervention aimed at effecting fundamental personality change in patients presenting with gross pathology, or psychiatric evaluation and/or treatment of individuals in whom the relationship of the character disorder to social/environmental factors is not always clear, can and should be augmented, if indicated, with services aimed at easing these patients' social situations as well as helping them to express feelings about the social dilemma in which emotional difficulties may be rooted.[13] In general, the author's work with this population supports the notion that the diagnostic skills of psychiatry are helpful in many or most cases, and that close collaboration and consultation between psychiatry and social work are most effective in the majority of cases. In those individuals who are unresponsive to insight-oriented treatment, psychiatric treatment is undoubtedly essential, with social work services serving in a supportive way.

RESTRICTION IN LIFE-STYLE AND THE ROLE OF THE FAMILY

> **Case Example 3:** Mr. S. was 56 years old, married, with three adult children. He had worked at a chemical refinery plant for 11 years and had plans to retire at the age of 62. In the past two years he had been in a series of accidents involving chemical spills and had experienced acute symptoms related to toxic exposure following these spills. His symptoms necessitated brief (3 week) periods of medical leave during which time he improved to the point of being able to return to work.
> Complaints on his visit to the occupational health clinic, which followed a 5

week medical leave after the most recent of four accidents, consisted of lingering (acute) symptoms, newly-acquired sensitivity to lower levels of exposure (experienced while driving past the plant), and recent onset of related symptoms on exposure to other environmental stimuli (house paint, traffic fumes, etc.). His affect was depressed, his wife doing most of the talking.

In the interview, conducted jointly with the physician, Mr. S. expressed fears about returning to the workplace: he was certain that he would continue to have more "accidents" and that if another one occurred he "would never make it." He spoke of being the object of ridicule from other workers who blamed him for the accidents. Concern expressed about the nature of his "illness" was continually interwoven with insistence that he was so "disabled" by his symptoms that he would never be able to work in an industrial setting again and, probably— because he lacked alternative training—never work again, period. His wife, an RN, expressed anger at the whole situation, demanding that the company be made to pay him total temporary workers' compensation benefits until the age of 62, when he could receive Social Security.

Initial work with the S.'s involved meeting them at the union hall (rather than the hospital), where Mr. S. was able to be more assertive and Mrs. S. less agitated. The social worker also met in consultation with the physician and union president regarding the most effective avenues for compensatory and retirement benefits for Mr. S. The S.'s were then able to recover enough emotional strength to participate in group treatment, where they discussed with other couples the effect of illness on family life, among other related issues.

Case Example 4: Mrs. L. is 34 years old, married, with no children. She has an advanced degree in a laboratory science. She came to clinic two years following a putative chronic exposure to workplace chemicals which she claimed caused her to develop intolerance to a host of environmental exposures, including detergents, house paint, perfume, etc. Her exposure having immediately preceded her marriage, she had been supported the last two years by her husband. During this time, she had involved herself with her new marriage and refurbishing a newly bought home; the latter "project" had been a "mixed bag." While occasionally rewarding, it was frustrating in the main due to her intolerance to household chemicals.

Ostensibly, her purpose in coming to the clinic was to receive "recommendations" from the physician as to appropriate vocational aspirations, now that she was convinced that she was unable to practice her former trade.

With the support of brief social work intervention, Mrs. L. and her husband elected to avail themselves of short-term, multi-family group treatment, where Mrs. L. played a leadership role, offering technical information to group members and openly discussing her frustrations and fears regarding re-entry to the workforce.

Often the life-styles of patients with MCS presenting for treatment have already become so restricted that patient and family alike experience a state of crisis, occasionally precipitated by the actual or imminent loss of work and source of income. In patients and families for whom the ability to work and earn a livelihood is not an issue, the unhappiness of the patient and the effect on homelife of the patient's condition, including the patient's inability to carry out traditional housework chores or other family obligations, may be the predominant source of strain.

Exploration of pre-morbid life-style patterns often reveals normal or quasi-normal behaviors that appear to have come to a gradual or abrupt stand-still with the onset of MCS. Attempts at interpreting the restrictive life-style behavior of MCS patients as a pattern in the overall patient and/or family dynamic, initially and even well into the treatment, should generally be avoided unless undertaken with extreme caution, as these attempts will almost invariably be met with resistance. Rather, one may offer psychological support and clarification of the role of "patient" and its effect on family functioning, encouraging ventilation and asking questions or commenting on inconsistencies and inappropriate emotions. The recommendation of further restrictions has not been shown to be effective, in fact it may be harmful.[12] Rigidity surrounding the physician's recommendation of alternative jobs "free from exposure," although reflecting the surface desire of MCS patients, may create further vocational adjustment problems. In fact, such restrictive recommendations may only reinforce personality traits (and/or disorders) that are part of the overall adjustment problem of patients in whom the syndrome of MCS develops.

> **Case Example 5:**   Mr. C. was awarded workers' compensation benefits for permanent partial disability resulting from MCS, after exposure to industrial solvents. He was referred for vocational rehabilitation for an exposure-free job, the training for which involved daily classroom instruction. After a period of a few weeks, he dropped out of the training program, explaining that he could not tolerate the odor of furniture polish used on the classroom desks. Following consultation with his physician, Mr. C. decided to take a job driving a bus, where he was exposed to diesel fumes but where he felt more at ease with his skills. He has remained at this job, making necessary adjustments to his chronic sensitivity symptoms, and seeing his physician every 3–6 months for psychological supportive treatment.

SUMMARY

Treatment of MCS, an illness characterized by reaction to a multiplicity of factors coming from within the patient and from the social and physical environment, must incorporate multiple types of help, all directed toward supplying what these patients require. Medical, psychiatric, and social work treatment are all significant and all different, with overlap in several areas. As in all practice in the medical setting, the overall function of the social worker is to enable the MCS patient to make use of what the physician has to offer by supporting the patient's capacity to cope with the social and emotional impact of his/her illness.

REFERENCES

1. Arndt R: Coping with job stress: The role of the union safety and health committee. Labor Studies J 5:53, 1981.
2. Bluestone B: The poor who have jobs. Dissent 15:410, 1968.
3. Cockerill E.: New emphasis on an old concept in medicine. *In* Kasius C (ed): Principles and

Techniques in Social Casework. New York, Family Service Association of American, 1950, pp 360–369.

4. Goldstein H: Starting where the client is. Social Casework 64:267, 1983.
5. Hollis F: The techniques of casework. *In* Kasius C (ed): Principles and Techniques in Social Casework. New York, Family Service Association of America, 1950, pp 412–426.
6. Karasek R: Jobs where stress is most severe (interview). U.S. News and World Report 95:45, 1983.
7. Margolis HM: The biodynamic point of view in medicine. *In* Kasius C (ed): Principles and Techniques in Social Casework. New York, Family Service Association of America, 1950, pp 349–360.
8. Nelson JC: Treatment of patients with minor psychosomatic disorders. Social Casework 50:581, 1969.
9. Reynolds B: Learning and teaching in the practice of social work. New York, Farrar and Rinehart, 1942, p 49.
10. Stewart DE, Raskin J: Psychiatric assessment of patients with 20th-Century disease (Total Allergy Syndrome). Can Med Assoc J 133:1001, 1985.
11. Tabor M: The stress of job loss. Occup H S 5:20, 1982.
12. Terr AI: Environmental illness: A clinical review of fifty cases. Arch Intern Med 146:145, 1986.
13. Towle C: Therapeutic criterial in social agencies. Am J Orthopsychiatry 9:399, 1939.
14. Tupper M: Personal communication.

MARK R. CULLEN, MD

MULTIPLE CHEMICAL SENSITIVITIES: SUMMARY AND DIRECTIONS FOR FUTURE INVESTIGATORS

THE PRESENT STATE OF THE ART

The contributions to this issue were solicited under the proviso, expressed in the introduction and to the authors, that its objectives were limited—not to proselytize the unconvinced with dogma but to share common uncertainty. My prior working presupposition was that too little could be widely enough agreed upon to allow development of more than a primitive research agenda; anything vaguely resembling concensus appeared inconceivable at the outset.

In fact, several common themes emerge recurrently in the reviews despite differences in focus, emphasis and perspective. The most important are these.

1. MCS patients suffer from a real and serious chronic disorder that cannot be dismissed trivially as a "normal" variation or the "low end" of a continuous distribution of host responses to irritant, odoriferous or intoxicating chemicals. Such explanations could never account for the intensity of clinical manifestation in many, the eclectic pattern of sensitivities in each (e.g., some patients can continue to smoke), nor the frequently abrupt onset of manifestations in mid-life, often after some sort of environmental "event."

2. MCS is a multifactorial disorder in which almost all experts agree psychological and psychosocial disruption are prominent features. Many reviewers also believe that one or more physiologic disruptions also occur either as predisposing, causal or associated phenomena, though biologic alterations and their importance relative to the conspicuous, widely acknowledged social and mental aspects remain highly controversial.

3. Treatment of MCS, though usually requiring initial avoidance of certain environmental substances, cannot be effectively managed by expanded or unlimited restrictions from exposure to "chemicals." In fact, a primary goal of all proposed therapy seems to be reduction in avoidance behaviors. This concept pervades the reviews and should dispel the popular misconception that environmental physicians and scientists, especially clinical ecologists, generally favor social and physical

From Yale New Haven Occupational Medicine Program, Yale University School of Medicine, New Haven, Connecticut

Reprint requests to Mark R. Cullen, MD, Occupational Medicine Program, School of Medicine, 333 Cedar Street, New Haven, CT 06510 isolation or scientifically arbitrary controls on chemical use as the solutions to the MCS problem.

Beyond these elements, however, lies a patchwork of conceptual frameworks, isolated and unconfirmed data, and an array of clinical anecdotes. It can hardly be a stylistic coincidence that most contributors and the editor offered case material in the places where some data would better fit! Nonetheless, taking the common ground as a point of embarkation and the controversy as grist, the elements needed to construct a serious and programmable research framework are largely at hand in the preceding pages. In the following sections, I shall outline those that seem reasonably well founded in existing data or theory, technically feasible, and *a priori* likely to answer major outstanding questions.

EPIDEMIOLOGY

The most immediate need is for expanded *descriptive* studies characterizing the clinical and demographic features of MCS and the populations from which they must (ultimately) be differentiated. Of particular interest would be studies with longitudinal data that may help elucidate the "natural" history of the illness as well as general patterns of response to more common social and clinical interventions. It is especially important that biases inherent in the choice to seek medical care, referral pattern, diagnostic label, and follow-up be recognized—avoided if possible but at least accounted for.

A very special possibility for descriptive study and one with potentially extraordinary heuristic value for investigations of its kind would be an attempt to ascertain historically if MCS or illnesses like it (however they may have been perceived) were described prior to the "chemical age" (which burgeoned between the World Wars). Evidence of a prevalent MCS-like disorder in the 19th century would weigh against a primary pathogenic role for certain chemicals *per se* and speak to other possibilities, including those raised in Dr. Brodsky's provocative essay.

However constructed, the goal of descriptive studies must be refinement of the diagnostic criteria, in particular the very tentative boundaries with other diagnostic entities such as allergic, anxiety, panic and post-traumatic stress disorders, and physiologic sequelae of CNS intoxication or injury, especially by organic solvents. In this regard it should be commented that the spectrum of solvent-related chronic sequelae are themselves far from well characterized and may well overlap with MCS.

On the analytic side, population studies are needed to elucidate factors which are associated with MCS and which might be causal. Needless to say, lest further confusion abound, such studies will require scrupulous attention to definitions and criteria for MCS and the related disorders. Perhaps these potentially invaluable types of investigations must await further descriptive work or, at a minimum, be linked to such efforts.

PATHOPHYSIOLOGY

Studies at several levels are needed to unravel this most central area of dispute. As with the epidemiologic agenda above, attention to definitions, avoidance of biases and careful selection of controls—which have vitiated much of the data presented in this volume—may be as crucial as investigational strategy in efforts designed to explicate disease mechanisms.

First, clinical studies comparing biological, psychological and sociological features of interest among MCS patients and appropriate controls will be needed, if only to sharpen existing hypotheses. Dr. Galland's study, though limited by retrospective design and therefore various clinical biases, would be an example of this. Such comparisons could define what if any reliable indices of biochemical, physiologic, immunological, microbiologic or even genetic abnormalities exist in MCS patients that distinguish them from normal subjects and individuals with the several related clinical disorders alluded to above. Similarly, differences in neurobehavioral function, chemistry or physiology could be demonstrated or excluded. Although these correlations could not in and of themselves prove that a particular associated finding is causal, absence of measurable differences would make such a relationship improbable.

A further refinement would be carefully controlled experimental challenges in the laboratory of patients and appropriate controls to predetermined doses of offending agents, observing both subjective and measurable physiologic responses. The problems of "masking" the challenges to assure true double-blinding raises technical difficulties that are not, I believe, insurmountable; the importance of blinding from a pathophysiologic perspective is obvious. If properly performed such experiments could provide very strong evidence for or against biological factors having a central pathogenic role in the hallmark clinical feature of the disorder—reactivity to low dose chemical exposures. Another exciting aspect of this approach is that it need not await the outcomes of epidemiologic or other observational studies, providing subjects and controls are thoughtfully selected and meticulously described.

A final approach that deserves mention is the possibility of developing an animal model of MCS by one or more interventions approximating the purported human experience, e.g., delivering repeated small doses of chemicals after an intoxicating "challenge" dose; direct induction of suspect nutritional deficiency, candidal or viral superinfection with coincident chemical exposures, and so forth. The experimental approach offers the possibility of exploring more clearly psychologic models as well, given the remarkable sophistication of neurobehavioral toxicology at this juncture; perhaps investigators in this area, trained to elucidate mechanisms, should become involved in conceptualization of both experimental and observational strategies for the study of MCS and sooner rather than later.

DIAGNOSIS AND TREATMENT

Given the apparently great economic impact in terms of both health services and lost productivity/income of each case and the perception, at least, that the problem is pervasive, controlled clinical trials of diagnostic and treatment strategies would probably be justifiable and surely would be the most impartial means to the truth. Unfortunately, such experiments would really require vastly more data and clearer concepts in characterization of the disorder and its boundaries, and a more advanced understanding of the pathogenesis of the disease. Otherwise we would soon find ourselves formally comparing antifungal therapy with psychotherapy or behavior modification with sublingual desensitization.

On the other hand, diagnostic and therapeutic approaches such as those described above by Drs. Cone, Schottenfeld, McLellan, Hessl and Lewis are being developed and tried. Careful observation and reporting, with due caution about inherent biases in the method, might help eliminate certain obviously irrational approaches and might continue to stimulate increasingly refined ideas among those treating and studying these patients. Indeed, such an inductive approach has certainly been invaluable in psychiatry and clinical medicine generally, often revealing results clearly enough to obviate expensive experiments. Candidly, the major limitations of this approach are the dangerously vested stakes in particular "answers" revealed by some investigators; this can only lead to bias and mistrust and undermine the scientific value of simple observations by all.

CONCLUSION

The health problems of workers who react to low levels of environmental pollutants and chemicals, increasingly reported and recognized in recent years, has posed a serious dilemma for health providers from a wide area of disciplines, including generalists, internists, family practitioners, allergists, psychiatrists, social workers, and frequently occupational physicians and nurses. The inability of these professionals to provide satisfactory care from the patient's perspective has led to the emergence of new and alternative clinical theories and approaches, challenging traditional views. Unfortunately, the success of these alternative approaches has also not been demonstrated, fueling an ever widening and hostile debate in which the patient is held hostage and virtually all clinicians are rendered impotent because of widely known intraprofessional disagreements.

In this volume, starting with more patients than cures and more questions than answers, I have attempted to frame a dialogue to include the theories, data and anecdotes of the major interested professional parties I could identify. The assumption was that each would make some contribution to a foundation on which subsequent work could build.

For my own part, I must confess a certain satisfaction that the state of the art is farther along than I had presumed it to be. Hopefully, the synthesis I have attempted above, in the form of a program for future research, will at least lead to more enlightened discussion if not to some efforts to design and conduct studies themselves.

INDEX

Page numbers of article titles are in **boldface** type.